Muscle Building Diet

2 Books Bundle - Strength Training Nutrition 101: Build Muscle & Burn Fat Easily...A Healthy Way Of Eating You Can Actually Maintain

+

Meal Prep Recipe Book: 50 Simple Recipes For Health & Fitness Nuts

By

Marc McLean

Table of Contents

Time to serve up the starter....

Strength Training Nutrition 101:

Build Muscle & Burn Fat Easily...A Healthy Way Of Eating You Can Actually Maintain

Introduction

I love food.

I really love it. I know you do too. The health and fitness industry doesn't seem to love it quite so much.

We're bombarded with advice on what we should be eating, how much we should be eating...and what we should be avoiding like an STI.

There are so many diets out there we can't keep up...Paleo, vegan, raw food, SIRT, Atkins, vegetarian, alkaline....I'll leave it there. We could be here a while otherwise. Every diet has its die-hard followers who insist their way is the only way. Not only does this do your head in, it also leaves you confused.

Maybe I shouldn't eat meat? Maybe carbs are the devil? Maybe I should be eating a garden full of greens for breakfast?

This book wasn't written to preach to you about any particular diet. In fact, I hate the word 'diet', I simply prefer a healthier way of eating. Diets are no fun – and most of them don't last.

With the title *Strength Training Nutrition 101*, I reckon you've figured this book is aimed at people who are fond of picking up a dumbbell or two. But I also want to make clear that I won't be regurgitating the usual "you MUST eat six small healthy meals per day" nonsense.

That's what we've heard from 95% of people in the health and fitness industry over the past decade and longer. I've read the same approach in several high profile fitness books and still see it in health magazines, as if it's the only proven way to develop muscle and keep your metabolism at a healthy level to stay lean too.

I tried that approach – eating/grazing every 2-3 hours - for way too many years. Guess what? It left me bloated, miserable and I felt like crap.

Then there's the chicken and broccoli brigade. You see it everywhere on Instagram, people cooking a week's worth of chicken and broccoli, placing it all neatly in 7 containers, and then uploading pictures of said 'prepped' cuisine.

F*ck eating the same old, boring, dry, tasteless chicken and soggy greens every day. Think I'd rather become one of those housebound 56 stone men you sometimes see on TV than live like that.

Here's a better idea: how's about we just eat as clean as possible Monday-Friday, limit sugar and booze, live a little more at the weekend, and actually go back to eating our meals in a more normal way?

We've made the uncomplicated way too complicated when it comes to diet and nutrition, particularly for weightlifters looking to gain muscle and strip fat. Want to transform your body and get in better shape? You don't have to go to crazy extremes.

Yes, protein builds muscle – but we don't really need 200, 300...or 400 grams per day like we read about in some fitness magazines. That's just insane.

Yes, energy drinks can give you a boost before your workout. Most of them also contain double the amount of sugar you should have in one day...with ridiculous amounts of caffeine too.

Yes, some supplements can assist in you hitting your health and fitness goals, but what about building a solid nutritional foundation first by eating plenty of whole foods?

The bottom line is that sticking with good nutrition should not be hard work. It should be easy to follow, manageable, and never actually feel like a 'diet'. Since I took up weight training as a ridiculously frail and pale 16-year-old back in 1998, I've experimented with countless ways of eating for energy, performance, muscle gain, keeping my bodyfat levels low and most importantly optimal health.

I've studied various nutritional courses, read countless books and articles, and used myself as a human guinea pig over the past 18 years in the quest for the best approach for all the goals I mentioned above.

The result? I have a formula for eating that is not only healthy, helps me hit all those health and fitness goals...and is <u>easy to maintain</u>. That's the key – if your diet is too complicated or restrictive then you're going to get pissed off in no time and will probably end up going bananas in the nearest Pizza Hut.

In Strength Training Nutrition 101, I share with you how to simplify the way you eat and my golden rules for clean eating. I also reveal my pre-workout nutritional approach that gives me bags of energy and maximises my effort in every workout.

Confused about what you should be eating and when after your gym sessions? I share advice to help you get the most out of all your hard strength training work.

As for supplements, there's so much out there that you could easily spend a fortune. You could also easily waste that fortune. There's a lot of unnecessary, and potentially dangerous, junk out there. You don't need to blow cash on supplements as a proper, healthy diet will give your body the tools it needs to repair, rebuild and remodel your body.

But there are still a handful of (all natural) healthy supplements that I include in my strength training regimen that are really effective. I share my recommended products with you towards the end of the book - and there's also a supplements guide bonus for you for buying this book.

Now onto the main course.

Chapter 1:

Simplifying Diet and Nutrition For More Muscle and Less Fat

If you're talking to your local gym instructor, personal trainer, or any bodybuilder/powerlifting pals then there's a fair chance they'll say: "Eat regular smaller meals throughout the day, with plenty of protein, that's the way to build and keep muscle."

See, that's the advice that's been spouted for years. Six smaller meals, some even munch through 7 or 8, going crazy for calories and ridiculous amounts of protein to build muscle mass. In fact, I know one bodybuilder who says he eats TEN smaller meals per day and he basically carries plastic tubs of food everywhere with him.

Surely we're verging on ridiculous when it gets to that stage? That just ain't natural. In fact, it's mental. Don't get me wrong, it DOES work for building muscle. I'm simply arguing that it's not the only way – and that there are a good few downsides to doing it.

You may have been trying to figure out how you're going to manage to prepare and devour so many meals in a day. You may already have been doing it. Prepping food every night or morning, eating by the clock, counting calories and grams of protein like some sort of macronutrients military exercise.

You can choose to do that each day. Every day. Or you can eat in what I consider a more normal way (3-4 meals per day) and still build a strong, athletic, lean physique. I'll also show how eating this way is highly effective for burning fat, while preserving muscle.

I followed the six smaller meals advice for the best part of a decade. Here's what happened...

It left me feeling bloated all the time.

The constant clock watching for scheduling meals was monotonous.

The endless food prepping made me want to chop my own head off.

I spent way too much time on the toilet.

I became a slave to my diet.

It was all way too stressful. But I still did it for those 10 years because I thought that was the only way to build muscle and stay in great shape. Looking back on it now, it was nuts.

I changed my mind around 2011, thanks to two people. Kettlebell and hormone optimisation expert Mike Mahler – and my old flatmate Ryan. My friend Ryan moved in with me after splitting up with his girlfriend and he was also into fitness. He also did some weight training and some mixed martial arts too.

Ryan was in great shape and his abs were always ripped. To the point where I considered evicting him. I figured he must train harder, eat better and get in even more protein than I was. So I watched what he was up to – and was pretty shocked.

- While I was stuffing my face with a high protein breakfast within 30 minutes of waking up, Ryan would regularly skip breakfast.

- While I would be munching constantly to cram in calories and protein, Ryan would go long periods between meals and still maintain muscle.

- While I was so strict with my diet and struggled to see my abs, Ryan would occasionally eat junk food and STILL have that damn six pack.

- While I ate all the time, Ryan ate when he was "hungry".

It didn't make any sense. I was the one being mega strict with my nutrition, timing my meals perfectly, a total slave to my diet, and was pretty miserable with it all. Ryan didn't bother with all of that – and was in better shape than me. I remember asking him: "When do you fit in your extra meals? Do you eat a lot when you're at work?"

He said: "No, I don't want to eat 6 or 7 times per day. I eat when I'm hungry and just make sure the food's as healthy as possible."

Around the same time I came across Mike Mahler, an American kettlebell and hormone optimisation expert. Mike follows a vegan diet, eats three or four times per day, and is built like a machine. He also goes against the standard regular smaller meals theory and backs this up through his extensive research on hormones. (Which we'll talk about shortly).

Mike Mahler and my friend prompted me to dig a bit deeper behind their success in staying strong and lean. I found they had the following in common:

- They would take longer stretches between their meals, maybe 5-6 hours. This optimised their hormones, particularly master hormone leptin and increased their insulin sensitivity. (I'll go into more detail on the importance of this later).

- They both managed to get enough calories in over the course of the day to maintain and build muscle. The bigger portion of these were post workout – the prime time for flooding the body with nutrients it needs to repair and build muscle.

- They didn't stress out about meal frequency.

So yeah, I'm going against the grain (pun fully intended) when it comes to the typical diet for men and women looking to gain lean muscle. First, let's talk about the reasons FOR eating 6,7,8 or more smaller meals per day...and then swiftly debunk them.

Main reason #1

"You need to keep supplying your body with calories and protein throughout the day or you will lose muscle."

A study carried out by 11 sports nutrition experts shows that meal frequency is actually irrelevant, as long as enough calories and the right macronutrients are consumed over course of the day.

Dr John Berardi is the founder of Precision Nutrition, who are world leaders in sports nutrition, and he is one of the most highly respected experts on diet and nutrition. He was part of this study and admitted that he too had initially thought that splitting up your daily food intake was the best approach. Dr Berardi said that early research indicated this would speed up the metabolism, help control the hormones insulin and cortisol, and better manage the appetite.

Following their detailed review in the Journal of the International Society of Sports Nutrition, the 11 experts concluded that as long as we eat the right foods in the right amounts, meal frequency is irrelevant. (Further details of this study and other research mentioned later can be found at the end of this book). You can either eat lots of smaller meals every few hours or you can eat a few big meals with bigger breaks in between. It's up to you.

Also debunking the 'eat frequently to maintain muscle' argument is the emergence of The Warrior Diet. Many thousands of people around the world – including big name athletes – are having huge success in sport and developing strong, ripped physiques by following this diet...which is the complete opposite to the eating six or more meals per day. The Warrior Diet, developed by sports scientist and former Israeli Special Forces member Ori Hofmekler, essentially involves fasting for up to 18 hours per day and then feasting at night.

This radical way of eating has been shown to ramp up fat burning, boost energy – while surprisingly preserving muscle mass. There are countless stories of people getting in the best shape of their lives by fasting, or eating very lightly during the day, and then cramming in most of their calories in the evening. This of course also reduces the need for mind-numbing food prepping and eating constantly throughout the day.

The Warrior Diet is followed by sporting superstars including MMA former world champion Ronda Rousey, DC Maxwell, two time women's Jiu-Jitsu world champion, and Pavel Tsatsouline, who basically introduced kettlebell training to the Western world back in 1998. Pavel says he has "better things to do than graze all day".

Main reason #2

"You can't get enough calories in to maintain and build muscle by eating fewer meals per day."

Calories are important, there's no denying that. If you regularly eat too many you'll pile on the pounds. If you don't eat enough you'll lose weight. We get it. There are a few different factors affecting your calorie requirements, but you can roughly figure out how many calories you need using this simple calculation:

Lose weight: bodyweight in lbs x 12 = total number of calories.

Maintain weight: bodyweight in lbs x 15 = total number of calories.

Gain weight: bodyweight in lbs x 17 = total number of calories.

We'll go into more detail about calorie consumption and your body's protein needs a bit later. But first, we're looking at getting in enough calories in just three or four meals rather than six or more. This is simply done in two ways - eating more at each meal and adjusting your diet to include some higher calorie foods. Increasing your intake of healthy fats is a good option as fat provides 9 calories per gram, while protein and carbs provide 4 calories (energy) per gram.

"But won't eating more fat make me fat?"

Not if you eat the right types is the short answer. 'Good' fats are found in fish, plant foods such as nuts, avocados and olives, eggs and dairy. When pulling together your shopping list at the top have foods like salmon, almonds, free range eggs, tuna, olive oil, coconut oil, coconut milk and butter.

There was a long-standing misconception that saturated fats are bad for you when in fact they play several important roles in the body including the manufacture of hormones, stronger bones, boosting the immune system and improved brain health. I go into more detail on healthy fats and which fats to avoid later.

Five Reasons Why 3-4 Meals Per Day Is Ideal

So, we've dealt why eating lots of smaller meals every day is not necessary for building and maintaining muscle. Sure, it works – but it can be stressful, difficult to maintain and leaving you feeling like you're chained to a fad diet. Here are five reasons for eating 3-4 meals per day like, erm, most people do.

#1 Taking longer stretches between meals optimises leptin (the master hormone) and keeps insulin sensitive.

Getting down to how diet affects our body at a core level is by looking at our hormones. Hormones are chemical messengers released into the blood which control the functioning of our brain and body. They are responsible for everything from mood and sex drive to physical performance and body composition.

Leptin is a powerful hormone produced in fat cells, which is in control of all other hormones in the body. Eating fewer meals optimises leptin. Eating often, especially with the wrong kinds of foods and in large amounts, causes leptin resistance. This can lead to problems with weight, particularly around the midsection.

Hormone optimisation expert Mike Mahler says that the best way to get out of leptin resistance is to give your body a break from eating large volumes of food often. For those trying to lose fat, sticking with two to three meals per day, with five to eight hours between meals, will give the body an opportunity to use stored bodyfat at energy. For people with lower bodyfat levels and looking to gain more muscle mass, four meals per day with about four hours between meals is a better option.

#2 To enjoy your food and avoid unnecessary stressing about diet.

The average person is only awake 16 hours per day so to manage at least six small meals per day you're gonna have to eat every 2.5 - 3 hours. Every day. Every week. This means always keeping an eye on the time to check when your next 'feed' is. It means disturbing your work to snack in the office, eating breakfast as soon as you can after waking up, munching when you're not even hungry, taking food 'on the go' whenever you're out and about, always thinking about what and when you're eating next...

Don't know about you but I'm stressed even reading all of that! How's about we relax and just enjoy three or four meals – when we're actually hungry - instead?

#3 To avoid constant crazy prepping.

When I used to follow the old six-meals-per-day advice I had an entire cupboard full of Tupperware. About 93 tubs of all shapes and sizes – and with countless lids that never seemed to fit. This was for all the 'prepped' small meals I would usually make at night or sometimes in the morning.

I must've wasted about 157.5 days of my life preparing my 'on the go' food. The tuna pasta that I would eat mid-afternoon in between lunch and dinner, or the protein smoothie I would have between breakfast and lunch to bump up the calories and keep feeding my muscle protein. I feared that if I missed a meal my biceps would somehow shrivel up!

One word - insane. Unless you've got your own personal chef, it's a nightmare to keep up with food prepping.

#4 To ease stress on your digestive system.

The length of time it takes to digest food varies from person to person and it also depends on what type of foods you're eating. In a media interview, Dr Anton Emmanuel, consultant gastroenterologist at University College Hospital in London, estimated that it takes 2-3 hours for a 600 calorie roast dinner to be broken down in the stomach before moving on through the small intestine, colon and eventually being excreted around 24 hours later.

Constantly bombarding our stomachs with food so frequently will inevitably lead to the digestive system struggling to keep up, food being backed up, and our gut health being badly affected as a result. All of this often results in common problems today such as constipation, wind, heartburn, and Gastroesophageal Reflux Disease (GERD).

#5 Spend less time on the toilet pan.

Quite often those people eating smaller meals will consume a considerably higher number of calories than is necessary to keep building muscle mass. Yep, more calories from good food sources, combined with proper weight training, does equal more muscle mass. It also equals more time in the bathroom when you overdo it so much.

Life's too short to be sitting on the toilet pan...straining...and wiping your ass 79 times per week! I spent 10 miserable years being a slave to my diet, and falling off and on the wagon trying to stick to six meals per day. I hated it but persisted because I thought it was the only way to maintain muscle.

It's not.

CHECKLIST

- Eating 6 or more small meals per day is not necessary for building muscle and keeping fat levels low.

- Meal frequency is a "matter of personal preference" – as long as sufficient calories and nutrients are being taken in over the course of the day.

- Taking longer stretches between meals helps optimise the master hormone leptin and insulin sensitivity, which makes the body more efficient at burning fat and building muscle.

- Eating in a normal fashion, i.e. 3-4 meals per day, rather than the typical bodybuilder approach has several benefits such as easing the strain on your digestive system and avoiding constant food prepping.

Chapter 2:

The 7 Golden Rules Of Clean Eating

Eating clean all the time is a pain in the @ss. I get it. That's exactly why I always recommend eating as healthy as possible Monday-Friday and then loosening up a little at the weekend...without going too nuts.

Eating 'clean' in the broadest sense means reducing the following as much as possible in your diet: ready meals, takeaways, sugary drinks and foods, and generally all processed junk. It also means staying well hydrated and making sure you're getting enough vitamins and minerals to give your body the right tools to keep you healthy and to support your strength training goals.

You could train like Rocky Balboa in the gym, but if your nutrition sucks then you're going to get nowhere. At the same time, you don't have to go to other extremes and follow a super strict diet to get in great shape and stay healthy. That'll only make you miserable and you'll eventually go on the rebound and end up on a 17 day junk food bender!

Seriously, if you want to make positive changes and get real results from your efforts in the gym then pay attention to the following Golden Rules of Clean Eating. Some of them may be stating the obvious, some might be completely new concepts to you. No matter where you're at health and fitness wise, these 7 steps will guide you towards great results.

If your diet hasn't been the best and you've got plenty of work to do, then here's a tip: introduce one positive habit per week. This is what I do with all clients who join my online personal training program. If we try to change everything at once it becomes overwhelming and makes you want to quit. If we focus on one positive habit per week, i.e. ditch fizzy drinks and replace them with water, then we can build upon each one and ultimately get awesome results at the end of the 12 week program.

Eat Clean Following These 7 Golden Guidelines

#1 Green is great

This means eating more vegetables and fruit. Stating the obvious here I know, but let's be honest - most of us don't eat nearly enough fruit and veg. Four or five servings per day is recommended to provide vitamins, minerals and a healthy source of carbohydrates. Try and include them with every meal.

#2 The white stuff ain't so great...

I'm talking about refined sugar. Excess sugar in our diets makes us fat and sick. Natural sugars from sweet fruits – yes. Fizzy drinks - complete no-no. We'll go into the problems of too much sugar in your diet, along with my tips and tricks to reduce it, in much more detail later.

#3 Cook fresh as much as possible

When buying the ingredients and preparing food yourself you know exactly what's going into your meals. No dodgy additives on the menu! I recommend investing in a vegetable steamer and blender. These are the two must haves in my kitchen. The steamer helps cook your vegetables lightly so that they retain their goodness. Boiling for too long, and even worse microwaving, remove the vitamins, minerals and enzymes from plant foods. Meanwhile, a blender is essential for making healthy protein shakes, either for breakfast or post-workout.

#4 Drink plenty of water

Men should shoot for around 3 litres per day, with women going for around 2.5 litres. Medics estimate that more than half of Americans are chronically dehydrated and this can lead to a multitude of health problems including headaches, weight gain, fatigue, joint pain and high blood pressure.

Weight training also causes water loss through sweating and, with our muscles being made up of 79% water, we require extra h2o to recover properly following a workout. Buy a sports water bottle and take it everywhere with you. To work, to the gym, when out walking the dog. Get into the habit of having water handy and staying hydrated. We're also usually dehydrated in the morning after sweating in our sleep. I drink a pint of warm water with the juice from half a lemon when I wake up as this improves digestion, boosts your immune system, cleanses your body, and reduces inflammation.

#5 Beware of the long ingredients list

You'll have heard the "saying too many cook spoil the broth". Well, too many ingredients usually spoil the food. If the ingredients list on the packaging is long this generally means the food has been filled with too many chemical flavourings, preservatives and additives, and is likely to be processed to the point where there is little nutritional value.

When you start seeing too many weird words you can barely pronounce then steer clear. Here are a few examples...Butylated Hydroxyl-anisole', Monosodium Glutamate, Propyl P-hydroxybenzoate. Say what?

.

#6 Limit salt

Usually listed as 'sodium' on packaging, be careful that there's not too much in what you're eating. The recommended daily allowance of salt is 6g – one teaspoon – per day to avoid health issues like high blood pressure.

#7 Ditch the microwave

Microwaves zap the life out of your food, robbing it of digestive enzymes, vitamins and minerals. Most pre-packaged ready meals for the microwave often have little nutritional value in the first place compared to a meal cooked with fresh ingredients.

And 7 Ways To Help You Stay On Track...

#1 Avoid the booze

Okay we know alcohol is bad for us, but so is all the junk food we eat afterwards. Hangovers lower our blood sugar, make us feel terrible...and we usually turn to the unhealthiest foods to try and feel better. Hungover people naturally crave sugar, fat and simple carbs as a quick way to raise their blood sugar levels. If you're getting on a wee bit like me, then you'll know that the hangovers don't hang around for one day any more!

#2 Cook double the amount of food for dinner

Then have another serving for lunch the next day. This is an easy healthy habit to get into. Cooking freshly-made healthy dinners regularly at home is the way forward for eating clean – and you can kill two birds with one stone by cooking plenty and munching on the rest for lunch the following day.

#3 Don't buy in junk food

Let's be honest, if there's a choice between the good and bad stuff in our cupboards we'll probably go straight for the chocolate, biscuits, potato chips etc first. If they're within easy reach then they're going to get devoured at some point. Just remove temptation by completely bodyswerving them at the supermarket. Buy in plenty of vegetables and fruit, and stock up on healthy snacks such as packets of nuts and raisins, hummus, and oatcakes and natural unsweetened peanut butter.

#4 Don't hit that 'snooze' button too many times

If you're always out of bed late and rush around in the morning then your diet will always suffer. It's hard eating clean when you've only got 30 minutes to get showered, dressed, brush your teeth, get to work...and then think about filling your belly. Set the alarm a bit earlier than normal, fly out of bed, make yourself a delicious dish, and start the day as you mean to go on.

#5 Get breakfast and lunch ready the night before

Here's another way to make sure you don't grab a takeaway breakfast or eat junk on the run...make a healthy breakfast shake the night before. I mentioned earlier that a blender is a must have item in my kitchen and one could improve your diet big time too. Just Google 'healthy smoothie recipes' or 'clean eating smoothie' to get plenty of shake ideas. You can then grab the shaker as you run out the door and drink that one the way to work, rather than swinging past a fast food drive thru for a greasy breakfast.

#6 Think about how crappy you'll feel afterwards

When you're drawn towards a mega munch of treats, sweets and fast food, then focus on how you'll feel afterwards. How do you usually feel <u>after</u> a splurge when you've been trying to eat clean? The guilt usually kicks in pretty quickly, doesn't it? And there's a fair chance you'll feel bloated, tired, maybe even a bit sick after a large fast food meal. When you're struggling with the temptation of junk food, first focus on this familiar not-so-good feeling that usually occurs after you go off the rails. It can help you stay on track.

#7 Cut yourself a bit of slack at the weekend

As I mentioned earlier in this chapter, focus on eating super clean Monday-Friday and then cut yourself a bit of slack at the weekend. Making the right food choices consistently is essential, but don't treat eating and nutrition like some sort of military exercise. It'll never work – as most fad diets prove in the long run. You'll only end up back at square one.

Get stuck into your favourite takeaway meal on a Saturday night with some wine. Or popcorn and some chocolate at the cinema. As long as you don't go overboard, you'll still be able to make progress in your health and fitness goals.

CHECKLIST

- **The 7 Golden Rules Of Clean Eating in a nutshell:**

  - **Eat more vegetables and fruit.**

  - **Cut right down on refined sugar, no more than 35g per day.**

  - **Cook fresh as much as possible.**

  - **Limit salt to no more than 6g per day.**

  - **Drink 2.5 to 3 litres of water per day (ideally include a pint with fresh lemon juice in that too).**

  - **Beware of foods with too many dodgy additives and preservatives, the names of which you can barely pronounce.**

  - **Ditch the microwave...it zaps the goodness out of your food.**

- **And 7 ways to stay on track with clean eating...also in a nutshell:**

  - **Avoid boozing as much as you can...it's only going to turn you into a junk eating monster.**

  - **Make double the amount of food when cooking a home-made dinner – then have another serving for lunch the next day.**

  - **Simply bodyswerve the junk food at the supermarket – because if it's in your cupboard you'll likely choose that before the healthy foods.**

  - **Get up bright and early so you're not rushing around in the morning and have time to make a** healthy breakfast and lunch.

-    Alternatively, make a healthy breakfast shake the night before, put it in a shaker and then grab it on your way out the door the next day.

-    Think hard about how crappy you'll feel after your junk food splurge – the more you do it the more it'll put you off.

-    Eat clean Monday-Friday and cut yourself some slack at the weekend for some treats.

Chapter 3:

The 'Poison' In Our Diets

Are you struggling to lose the flab around your waist?

annoyed at the lack of muscle definition?

fed up eating tasteless 'low fat' foods – while not actually losing much fat?

do you lack energy and catch every cold, infection, virus that is floating around?

Cutting back on sugar might well be the answer to your problems. Too much refined sugar on a daily basis will play havoc with your body – and prove to be a roadblock to getting in great shape and achieving optimal health. In fact, it's often considered a POISON to the body. Rewind to 1957 and Dr William Coda Martin first classified refined sugar as a poison because it is depleted of its life forces, vitamins and minerals when processed from sugar cane plants.

He said: "What is left consists of pure, refined carbohydrates. The body cannot utilise this refined starch and carbohydrate unless the depleted proteins, vitamins and minerals are present."

Fast forward to 1972, British physician and endocrinologist John Yudkin wrote the book *Pure, White and Deadly* warning of a health disaster due to the increase in consumption of sugar in our Western diets. And these days...

- Refined sugar contributes to around 35 million deaths around the world, according to researchers at the University of California. They commented in the journal Nature that it should be considered as toxic as tobacco and alcohol.

- Cancer, heart disease, diabetes, metabolic syndrome and a multitude of other diseases have been strongly linked with over-consumption of refined sugar.

- Childhood obesity is at record levels in the US, UK and in many countries across Europe where processed, junk foods fill most space on supermarket shelves.

- The UK government came under more pressure in October 2005 to introduce a 'sugar tax' due to its links with obesity and links to illnesses such as diabetes. This came after new stats show that one in five children in the UK are obese by the time they leave primary school.

- In the US, the number of people who had diabetes due to chronic blood sugar issues saw an "alarming" rise from 26 million in 2010 to 29 million in 2014, according to the Centers for Disease Control and Prevention.

Think I've made my point. Not only is sugar directly linked to diseases such as cancer and heart disease, it weakens the immune system and robs your body of essential vitamins and minerals needed for a strong, healthy body.

How Excess Sugar Makes Us Fat

Too much glucose is the first issue. Whenever we fill our bodies with too much fuel, which is very easy with high sugar foods, the liver runs out of storage capacity. The excess sugar is then converted into fatty acids and is then returned to the bloodstream. This is then stored as bodyfat in your belly, hips, chest...and generally most places you don't want it.

The second issue is excess insulin. Insulin is a key hormone in the body, and is released in high amounts whenever you eat or drink a "simple" carbohydrate, which includes the likes of white bread, white rice, baked white potato, bagels, croissants, cornflakes, cake, sugary drinks, beer, and anything that has high fructose corn syrup on the nutritional label.

When insulin levels are spiked the body's fat burning process is shut down so that the sugar that's just been consumed can be used for energy straight away. Sugar is shuttled into your muscles but, as soon as the muscle energy stores are full, the excess sugars are converted and stored as bodyfat. There are many ways you can drastically cut back on sugar in your diet and I'll share 10 simple ways you can start doing so today. First, here's a quick breakdown of different types of sugar.

- Sucrose – comes mainly from sugar cane or sugar beets.

- High fructose corn syrup (HFCS) – not technically a sugar, it is a liquid sweetener made from corn introduced to our diets in the 1970's.

- Fructose, maltose and dextrose – comes from fruits and starchy plants.

- Lactose – comes from dairy products.

Sugars consumed in large amounts contribute to obesity and disease, but the first two above are the real problem. Cane plants are stripped of all vitamins and minerals when refined to make common white sugar. In this state, it is considered toxic to the body by medical experts. Meanwhile, HFCS is an industrial food product which is far from natural.

The American Heart Association recommends that 37.5grams (around 7 teaspoons) of added sugar is the daily limit for men, while 25g (around 5 teaspoons) is enough for women. One 330ml can of Coke contains 35 grams alone. Be aware that there's likely too much sugar in your foods if sugar is listed close to the top of the ingredients list. Also, sugar is not always listed as sugar. Look out for the names of its man-made dodgy cousins including high fructose corn syrup, dried cane syrup and brown rice syrup. If there are several of them in the one food item then I'd steer clear.

10 Simple Steps To Reduce Sugar In Your Diet

#1 One lump, not two

Have one sugar in your tea or coffee instead of two. Then cut back on the number of cups of tea/coffee you have every day...and gradually wean yourself off the sugar.

#2 Super Stevia

Even better, use Stevia. It is a 100% natural zero calorie sweetener with numerous health benefits. Studies have shown that Stevia can actually reduce blood pressure and fight type II diabetes.

#3 Go herbal

Try out herbal teas instead of tea, coffee or soda. Herbal teas are awesome, with lots of varieties that are full of flavour and decaffeinated too.

#4 Let the fizzy drinks fizzle out.

If you drink juice/soda throughout the day gradually cut back by swapping some for a cup of water instead. Wean yourself off the fizzy drinks gradually by replacing it with water instead.

#5 Change up your breakfast.

Do you eat cereal for breakfast? Most have high levels of sugar (Up to three teaspoons per small 30g bowl). So why not swap cereal for porridge or wholegrain toast with scrambled eggs?

#6 Ditch the desserts.

If you have desserts after dinner or chocolate most nights then gradually cut that out one day at a time.

#7Add spices to your foods.

Cinnamon, ginger, nutmeg and cardamom will naturally sweeten your foods and reduce cravings for sugar.

#8Don't buy sugary snacks.

The cravings will come and go for chocolate and other sweet foods, but if you don't have these snacks within easy reach in your house or work office then you will be able to cut down on sugar intake.

#9Have a piece of fruit instead.

This can help satisfy sugar cravings and the natural sugars fruit contain are healthier than refined sugars.

#10Read the labels.

Sugar is not always listed as sugar. Look out for names including high fructose corn syrup (remember than one?), dried cane syrup, sucrose and brown rice syrup. These can all be listed as separately on ingredients lists, and if the names are listed close to the top there is probably a considerable amount of sugar in the food.

Did the sugar message get through? Was all the chat about cancer, heart disease, diabetes and general doom as delightful and uplifting as I intended? Good - job done. Let's be honest, you (probably) won't drop dead after the next king size Mars bar you eat. But if you want to be healthy and are serious about getting in good shape then cutting out as much sugar as possible is a massive step.

Remember, excess sugar turns to fat – and both refined sugar and high fructose corn syrup are the worst offenders. Doesn't mean that you don't have to give up treats forever. Just follow the 10 steps above and gradually cut back your sugar intake overall.

CHECKLIST

- Refined sugar is considered a poison in many medical circles and has been directly linked to various killer diseases including diabetes, cancer and heart disease.

- Glucose overload from too much sugar results in the liver converting it into fatty acids. These are then returned to the bloodstream and stored as bodyfat.

- Excess sugar also causes our insulin levels to spike and, when our muscle energy stores are full, it is also stored as bodyfat.

- Look out for other forms of man-made sugars listed as high fructose corn syrup, dried cane syrup and brown rice syrup on food labels. Steer clear if there are several of these names on the packaging.

- Choose some, or all, of these options to reduce your sugar intake:

  - Cut down on the sugar in your tea or coffee.

  - Better yet, drink herbal teas.

  - Choose natural sweetener Stevia instead of sugar.

  - Ditch desserts after dinner.

  - Replace fizzy drinks with water.

  - Add spices to your foods for more flavouring.

  - Don't buy in sugary snacks, there are healthier alternatives like fruit.

  - Read food labels and keep an eye out for high sugar content.

Chapter 4:

Making The Right Food Choices

Building muscle is not all about how much protein you eat. Losing fat is not about how much fat you eat. And carbohydrates are not all bad, despite all sorts of new 'low carb' or 'carb cycling' diets we hear about these days.

Diet and nutrition can get crazily complicated in the health and fitness industry. Fad diets, calorie counting, macronutrients calculations and fancy supplements. But the bottom line is that you won't gain lean muscle or be able to strip fat effectively if you don't get the basics of making correct food choices right. Our macronutrients are of course split into three categories: protein, carbs and fats. Each macronutrient can also be split into two more groups…the good guys and the bad guys.

Yep, the *sources* of your carbs, protein and fat are what's most important. Brown rice is high in carbs...but so is white bread. Deep fried chicken is high in protein and fat...so are almonds. Which will you choose? Let's take each of the three macronutrients and sort the good from the bad.

Carbohydrates

Carbs are the body's main source of fuel and it's a straight up battle between complex (the good guys) and simple (bad) carbs. Complex carbohydrates are unprocessed and contain the fiber found naturally in the food, while refined carbs have been processed and had the natural fiber stripped out.

Simple carbohydrates are made up of easy to digest sugars with little nutritional value for your body. The higher in sugar, the worse the carbohydrate is for you. Obviously cookies, sweets and desserts are among the worst offenders – but you can still enjoy them occasionally.

A much better option is for your daily intake to be made primarily made up of complex carbohydrates. Dietitians and nutritionists compare carbohydrate foods based on their glycemic index. This basically refers to how quickly and how high your blood sugar will rise after eating carbohydrates. Lower glycemic foods are healthier and most, but not all, complex carbs fall into this category.

The Goodfellas: sources of complex carbs include: vegetables, fruits, wholegrains, brown rice, beans, legumes, nuts and seeds. Fill up on these.

The Bad Guys: common simple carbohydrate foods include: cakes and cookies, pastries and desserts, white breads, white pasta, white rice. Limit these.

Protein

Protein's main role is for tissue growth and repair. Forget building muscle without a decent supply of protein. But how much protein do we need exactly? That's something we'll delve deeper into later. First, let's break protein down. Protein is made up of 'amino acids', which are the building blocks of the body for repairing and developing muscle. They also play a role in energy, weight loss, and brain function. Of the 20 amino acids, there are nine 'essential' ones, which the human body cannot produce.

What should be on the menu to build muscle? Food sources considered 'complete proteins' – meaning they contain all nine essential amino acids - or a combination of 'incomplete proteins' to ensure you cover all bases. Complete proteins are primarily animal-based foods and a few plant-based sources. These include: meat, poultry, fish, dairy products, eggs, quinoa, buckwheat, hemp seeds.

Have you Googled those last two already? No, they're not on my shopping list either. And don't panic if you're a vegetarian or vegan. You can still grab all essential amino acids and build muscle by feasting on a variety of incomplete protein sources including nuts, seeds, grains and vegetables. There are also some awesome plant-based protein supplements, such as brown rice protein and vegan blend protein, that I switched to years ago.

Personally, I avoid red meat and don't eat much animal protein at all, apart from chicken 3-4 days per week. My body finds it harder to digest meat and I believe there's truth in the arguments that too much animal protein is bad for our health. I'm not trying to convince you either way, I'll leave it up to you to do your own research.

Fats

Fat clogs your arteries. Fat makes you fat. Fat causes obesity. Fat started World War Two...I reckon fat gets a pretty bad rap. For decades the medical establishment had us believe that fat is at the root cause of our health problems. *'Eat a low fat diet and you will lose weight,'* they told us. *'Cut down on fat for better health,'* they promised.

Fact: The 'low fat' diet was first recommended to Americans back in 1977 – yet obesity has more than doubled since then.

Fact: The standard Mediterranean diet is as high as 40% fat, yet research has shown it cuts the risk of heart disease and strokes by around a third.

Fact: Eating those Satanic saturated fats, that we have been told we must avoid, is the best way to reduce a substance called lipoprotein – which is strongly linked to heart disease.

Just like carbs, there are good guys and bad guys when it comes to fat. There are four main types of fat: saturated (good), monounsaturated (good), polyunsaturated (okay, but when heated we have a problem) and trans-fats (bad).

Here's how I sum the whole situation up:

- Saturated fats are better for us than we were led to believe.

- Trans-fats (aka man-made ones) are to be avoided like the plague.

- Monounsaturated are good for us.

- Polyunsaturated fats are okay in moderation.

The Goodfellas: fish, unrefined animal fat, plant foods such as nuts, seeds, olives and avocados, eggs and dairy, olive oil, coconut oil etc. Get stuck into these.

The Bad Guys: fried foods, baked goods, margarine, and processed snack foods. I've also lumped vegetable oils (such as sunflower, corn, canola etc) in with the bad guys, but there is still debate about whether or not they're good for us. I err on the side of caution. Limit or eliminate these.

"Aren't saturated fats bad for us?...."

I can hear some readers saying this already. There's still plenty of debate over saturated fats, but it seems health experts are finally catching up to the idea that added sugars are public enemy #1, with dodgy man-made trans-fats (used in the likes of vegetable oil and margarine) also culpable. Plenty of leading medical researchers and top health and fitness experts, including the hugely-respected Charles Poliquin and Mark Sisson, have long argued the case that saturated fats are not only good for us, but they play some really important roles in the body.

Mark Sisson, of Mark's Daily Apple, recommends saturated fats in animal products and the likes of extra virgin olive oil as part of a healthy diet. He often writes about their importance in immune function, enhancing calcium absorption and providing fat soluble vitamins. The late Mary Enig PHd, nutritionist and researcher, had been screaming about how we had it all wrong on saturated fats for years. She spent decades studying the role of fats in the diet and disputed the widely held medical views that high levels of saturated fats caused heart disease.

Enig, who was awarded Master of the American College of Nutrition, argued that foods high in natural saturated fats, such as butter & coconut oil, are *beneficial* for heart health. *She wrote: "The much-maligned saturated fats—which Americans are trying to avoid—are not the cause of our modern diseases. In fact, they play many important roles in the body chemistry. The scientific evidence, honestly evaluated, does not support the assertion that 'artery-clogging' saturated fats cause heart disease."*

The American Heart Association still advises us to limit saturated fats, arguing that studies have shown it increases level of 'bad' cholesterol. Some other medical experts still believe too much saturated fat contributes to heart disease. I'm in the pro-saturated fat camp and reckon fats make up around 30%-40% of my diet. My main sources are butter, nuts and coconut milk.

Eating For Your Body Type

Food provides us with fuel and the nutrients needed for repair, growth and development. So how much protein, carbs and fats should someone involved in strength training be taking in to gain lean muscle and keep bodyfat low? The Institute of Medicine calculated an acceptable macronutrient distribution range for active people as: carbohydrate (45%-65%), protein (10%-35%), and fat (20%-35%).

Our bodies are different so there's no perfect ratio of macronutrients that applies to everyone, but by figuring out our body type we can get a fair idea of how to mix up our carbs, protein and fat. *Ectomorph, mesomorph* and *endomorph* body types each have different metabolic rates and hormonal responses to food. I was a 100% ectomorph (aka super skinny) before I took up weight training, but I'd say I'm more between ectomorph and mesomorph now that I've managed to gain and retain muscle mass due to years of training.

Ectomorph

This is the 'hard gainer' body type. Naturally slimmer people who have a faster metabolism and a higher tolerance for carbs. They can eat more junk food than most and generally get away with it. Their typical macronutrients split could be: carbs 55%, protein 25%, fats 20%.

Mesomorph

The people skinny and heavier dudes love to hate. They have a naturally athletic physique with more muscle mass and seem to get in great shape with less effort. Moderate carbs with higher ratio of protein and fats. Typical ratio would be: carbs 45%, protein 35%, fats 20%.

Endomorph

People with these body types pack on muscle with ease, but have a bigger, rounder frame and can struggle to lose weight. Their diet should have fewer carbs, with more protein and healthy fats. Typical ratio – carbs – 35%, protein – 35%, fats – 30%.

These are just averages and the ratios can be adjusted depending on the particular goal at the time. For example, an endomorph who wants to lose weight might cut carbs down further to 10-15%, bump up the number of protein foods, and add a few more healthy fat food sources. Or a mesomorph, who is neither fat nor thin but is looking to develop a six pack, might also cut carbs so that the body turns to fat stores for energy.

Whatever category you fall into, or if you're split between two, adjust your protein, carbs and fats to suit. If you're overweight and have a bigger frame, it would make sense to lower your carbs intake, while if you are too skinny you can take in more regularly to help add on some weight.

- Carbohydrates: more of the 'complex' variety, less of the 'simple' ones. Fill up on vegetables, fruits, wholegrains, brown rice, beans, legumes etc.

- Protein: meat, poultry, fish, dairy products, eggs and plant-based foods such as quinoa, buckwheat and hemp seeds are all good sources.

- Fat: avoid trans-fats (fried foods, margarine etc) as much as you can. Instead, get your fat fill from fish, unrefined animal fat, coconut oil, olive oil, plant foods such as nuts, seeds, olives and avocados, eggs and dairy.

CHECKLIST

- Carbohydrates are the body's main source of energy and are split into two types: 'complex' (the good guys) and 'simple' (the bad guys).

- Best carbohydrate sources: vegetables, fruits, wholegrains, brown rice, beans, legumes, nuts and seeds. Fill up on these.

- Worst carbohydrate sources: cakes and cookies, pastries and desserts, white breads, white pasta, white rice. Limit these.

- Protein builds muscle as one of its main roles is tissue repair and growth. Protein is made up amino acids which complete this process.

- Excellent protein sources: meat, poultry, fish, dairy products, eggs, quinoa, nuts, seeds, plant-based protein powder supplements.

- Not all fats are bad for us and, despite years of misinformation about saturated fat being unhealthy, it's argued now that saturated fat plays important roles in our bodies such as boosting the immune system, the manufacture of hormones and strengthening bones.

- Excellent fat sources: fish, unrefined animal fat, plant foods such as nuts, seeds, olives and avocados, eggs and dairy, olive oil, coconut oil.

- Fat sources to avoid: fried foods such as fries, crisps, cakes, margarine, processed snack foods, vegetable oils such as sunflower, corn, and canola.

- The 'ectomorph' naturally slimmer body type has a higher metabolism and a higher tolerance for carbs. Their typical macronutrients split would be around: carbs 55%, protein 25%, fats 20%.

- The 'mesomorph', aka naturally athletic body type, would eat roughly around: carbs 45%, protein 35%, fats 20%.

- The 'endomorph' bigger, rounder frame which adds muscle easily should have fewer carbs. Their typical ratio would be around: carbs – 35%, protein – 35%, fats – 30%.

Chapter 5:

Calories

So here's the deal: I'm not going to bang on about calories and insist you start counting them at every meal, every day, every week. That would make life pretty sh*t. And I don't want you turning into some sort of Rain Man mathematician as a side effect of trying to get in great shape.

BUT...I'm going to be straight up and tell you that calories are rather important when it comes to hitting your health and fitness goals. Bottom line is: if you don't take in enough calories you've got no chance of building muscle, and if you're trying to lose weight and develop lean muscle then you're going to have to be in a calorie deficit for a period.

A kilocalorie (kcal), better known as calorie, is a measure of the amount of energy in our food. It supplies our body with fuel to get through the day, our activities, our workouts etc. If we regularly take in more than we expend we gain weight – and vice versa. When clients first come to me and tell me their fitness goals, one of the first questions I ask them is: *"Do you know roughly how many calories you take in each day?"*

I've yet to meet a single client who does. And that's cool because who wants to be tracking numbers all the time when we're enjoying our food? But when we've got a particular fitness goal to hit it helps us get there much sooner when we know our calorie numbers. When you reach your ideal weight/size level you don't have to be as precise, but it's still really beneficial to know *roughly* how many calories you should be taking in on an average day, and a *fair idea* of how many calories are in your meals.

It's not as boring as it sounds because once you've been tracking calories for a little while, you soon learn roughly how much is in most of the common foods you eat. For me personally, I hover around 2,300-2,700 calories per day to maintain muscle and stay at the same weight. If I eat less than 2,000 calories per day for a week or more then I lose weight.

Most people looking for support from me are overweight and want to lose weight and develop muscle. We reduce their daily calories, along with a strength training program, to focus primarily on dropping the excess bodyfat. Then we'll make calorie adjustments and continue lifting weights to develop muscle. If a slim person comes to me saying they struggle to gain even a single pound of muscle, we'll bump up their calories along with implementing a weight training program consisting mainly of compound exercises as described in my book *Strength Training Program 101: Build Muscle & Lose Fat...In Less Than 3 Hours Per Week.*

A Simple Formula For Working Out Your Daily Calorie Requirements

How many calories we require each day depends on various factors including sex, age, height, weight, and activity levels. But without getting too complicated and trying to make it a perfect science, there's actually a simple calculation for figuring out roughly how many calories an average active person requires. How many calories should you be consuming? Do the math...

<u>Maintenance:</u> *Bodyweight in lbs x 15 = number of calories*

<u>Weight gain:</u> *Bodyweight in lbs x 17 = number of calories*

<u>Fat loss:</u> *Bodyweight in lbs x 12 = number of calories*

Therefore the sums for 160lb guy aiming to gain weight and size while building muscle would shoot for around 2,700-2,800 calories (160 x 17 = 2,720). Or a 170lb woman looking to lose fat would aim for around 2,000 calories per day (170 x 12 = 2,040).

These equations are effective guidelines for each goal will and keep you right when it comes to calories. But they aren't set in stone and can be adjusted slightly as you progress. For example, I'm a hard gainer who struggles to put on muscle mass. If I really wasn't seeing much progress after a few weeks I might actually increase multiplying my bodyweight from 17 to 18.

Someone determined to lose fat might multiply their bodyweight by 11 instead of 12 to reduce their calories a bit further. By adjusting calories as necessary, making the right food choices, and lifting weights regularly you'll be well on track to hitting your targets and seeing real changes in your body.

Building Muscle and Losing
Fat - Simultaneously

Muscle gain and fat loss – at the same time. It can be done. We know we need <u>sufficient calories to gain muscle</u> and a <u>calorie deficit for burning fat.</u>

We also know now how to work out roughly how many calories we need based on our personal goals. Calories are key to everything going to plan...but we don't just get them from the food and drink that passes our lips that day. We can also turn to stored bodyfat - which are essentially stored calories – to fuel our workouts and muscle building efforts. Whenever there's a calorie deficit the body will turn to fat stores for energy. If you're using that energy to lift heavy weights in the gym then we're getting 2 for the price of 1 here...losing excess fat in order to build muscle.

Going back to the example from earlier about the 170lb woman trying to lose fat. We worked out that she should be consuming around 2,000 calories per day to achieve this. Her maintenance calories including exercise should have been around 2,500. Where will her body get the missing 500 calories needed for energy and to build muscle? By burning bodyfat. There are roughly 3,500 calories in a pound of fat. 500 calories times 7 days amounts to 1 full pound of bodyfat being lost while fuelling muscle development.

A Top Tool For Tracking Calories...And Optimising Your Diet

The 'MyFitnessPal' app does everything – apart from shouting "don't eat that!!" – to optimise your diet and keep track of your calories. It's free to download on the iTunes and Android app stores and I use it with all my online personal training clients.

Calculating your calorie targets? Working out how much protein/carbs/fat you're taking in? Saving regular foods and recipes? Even scanning the barcodes of your food packets? This amazing app does it all for you. It's straightforward to use and will help you hit your health and fitness goals more easily. There are also demonstration videos for the app on YouTube for anyone who finds using it a bit tricky at first.

CHECKLIST

- A kilocalorie (kcal), better known as calorie, is a measure of the amount of energy in our food. It supplies our body with fuel to get through the day, our activities, our workouts etc.

- If we regularly take in more calories than we expend we gain weight – and vice versa.

- You don't have to count every single calorie, but if your fitness goal is to lose weight or gain weight then you should have a fair idea of your average calories in and out each day.

- The simplified calorie formula:

  Maintenance: *Bodyweight in lbs x 15 = number of calories*

  Weight gain: *Bodyweight in lbs x 17 = number of calories*

  Fat loss: *Bodyweight in lbs x 12 = number of calories*

- Whenever there's a calorie deficit the body will turn to fat stores for energy. If you're using that energy to lift heavy weights in the gym then it's 2 for the price of 1...losing excess fat in order to build muscle.

- Want the simple answer to tracking calories and monitoring your nutrition? Download the MyFitnessPal app and set up a free account.

Chapter 6:

Do We Really Need ALL That Protein?

The world's gone a bit mental for protein. People who barely exercise are drinking protein shakes these days, you can buy Weetabix 'Protein' in the supermarket, and I'm pretty sure I saw a Protein Mars bar in a shop the other day. WTF?

People who do strength training generally end up pretty obsessed by protein. Eggs for breakfast, chicken for dinner, protein shake straight after training. What goes with it...whether it's wholegrain bread, vegetables, pasta...is usually an after-thought. We're usually too busy trying to figure out yet another way to cook our chicken breast first.

But is it really necessary? Do we really need ALL that protein?

Turns out we don't – and it took me the best part of 15 years (and 4,093 cans of tuna) to realise it. That's why this entire chapter is dedicated to debunking the myth that you need massive amounts of protein to maintain or build muscle. This book cost less than the price of a tub of protein powder and if I'd known years ago what I know now I would have saved a fortune on food and supplements. This chapter alone could save you $$$$ too – and possibly even your health.

I've heard stories of personal trainers telling women to eat 180g, 200g or more of protein per day while doing strength training. These 125lbs women are loading up on eggs, bacon, whey protein shakes...struggling to get through it all each day to hit their protein targets. Then they're surprised when they're bloated, farting like mad, and are constantly constipated. Let's put that kind of protein intake into perspective....

Arnold Schwarzenegger, the world's greatest ever bodybuilder, weighing 220lbs, standing, 6ft 2 ins tall, only consumed around 150g of protein. This was when he was competing for the Mr Olympia title – which he won seven times. Meanwhile, these women are eating MORE protein than him - it doesn't make one bit of sense. We all know that protein builds muscle....but, again, do we really need ALL that protein?

I did a lengthy amount of research on this topic because, let's be honest, there's so much advice out there on diet, nutrition, supplements, macronutrients, micronutrients....that sometimes it makes you just wanna eat pizza and tell the health and fitness world to f*** off. I was really surprised about what I discovered and it appears that some protein myths that have been spouted by 'experts' and the multi-billion dollar protein supplement industry for decades.

You might choke on your protein shake while reading this but what if someone told you that....

- You could probably cut your protein intake by half – and still build and maintain muscle.

- One of the world's most famous bodybuilders only ate 60g of protein per day.

- An athlete who was consuming 300g of protein per day was shocked to discover most of it was going to waste...and he was developing worrying health problems as a result.

- Calories are a bigger factor when it comes to building muscle than you would believe.

- Our bodies can actually recycle amino acids themselves, meaning there is less need for a constant high supply of protein.

When it comes to building muscle and developing a strong, lean physique, the vast majority of experts in the health and fitness industry will tell us: "Eat more protein. Eat more protein…then have another plateful of protein." We're told to simply increase our protein numbers, train hard…and the muscle will come. The standard advice dished out by bodybuilders is: "You need 1g of protein per 1lb of bodyweight."

Some adverts in health and fitness magazines (which get paid megabucks for adverts by protein supplements companies funnily enough...) tell us we need as much as 300g or 400g to build maximum muscle. So while we're trying to cram in the equivalent of 10 x chicken breasts, or 12 cans of tuna, or 8 protein shakes, maybe it's worth asking who actually came up with these numbers anyway?

This more protein = more muscle idea seems too simplistic. Two very important factors are often ignored/forgotten about...

Protein *absorption* - a healthy digestive system can properly process the foods we eat to provide energy, extract the nutrients to nourish our cells, and help to build and repair muscle. Problem is, a high percentage of people living in the Western world don't have healthy digestive systems due to the processed junk that fills our supermarket shelves. The fact that the treatment of heartburn, constipation etc is a multi-billion dollar industry in America is proof of this. Many of us also live highly-stressed lives, and in times of stress our digestive system basically shuts down as our bodies go into 'fight or flight' mode. This means we don't break down food as we should - and certainly can't cope with ridiculous amounts of protein in those situations.

Secondly, the protein *source* is also an important factor. There are countless high protein foods we can choose from, but they are not all equal in nourishing the body and building muscle. For example, steak is one of the highest sources of protein and also contains a good dose of iron and creatine that you won't find in most other foods. It's hugely popular with bodybuilders - but takes up to 72 hours to be properly digested in the body.

It's not unusual for some bodybuilders to eat steak every other day in an attempt to keep building muscle. While the body is still processing the last one, along with other meals in between, it's looking highly likely that we're going to have some backing up of food. The body struggling to keep up is when digestive problems occur and toxins floating around in the body as a result can also lead to other health issues such as skin problems.

Is All That Extra Protein Going To Waste?

But how can we know for certain either way? How much of all that protein is actually being utilised by the body? <u>Not much</u> – is the answer from Dr Ellington Darden. After carrying out a unique two month-long protein study on himself back in 1970 and finding startling results, Dr Darden insisted that *"the biggest misconception 20 years ago, and still the biggest misconception today"* is the idea that we need huge people lifting weight need a huge amount of protein to build and maintain muscle.

This isn't the opinion of just another "fitness expert". Dr Darden was honoured by the President's Council on Fitness, Sports and Nutrition as one of the top ten health leaders in the United States. Back in 1970, as a competitive athlete and bodybuilder for around 20 years he was consuming 380g of protein per day. Half of this came from protein powder and he was also popping all sorts of nutritional pills to aid his muscle growth.

That was until one of his colleagues, Dr Harold Schendel Professor in the Food and Nutrition Department at Florida State University, told him that was way too much protein and he was wasting his time. Determined to prove he was right, Dr Darden set up a detailed study on his own body. For two months, he kept precise records of his dietary intake, of energy expenditure, and his general well-being. All his urine was collected and analyzed by a graduate research team in nutrition science.

The results? The study showed his body was excreting large amounts of water soluble vitamins, proteins and other nutrients. As he had been consuming massive doses for years, his liver and kidneys had apparently grown excessively large to handle the influx of all these nutrients.

Why You Need Less Protein Than You Think

If you've been lifting weights for a while I'm guessing you're devouring tons of high protein foods like steak, chicken, eggs, whey protein shakes etc. We work so hard to build the muscle that we want to make sure we make the most gains afterwards. We even watch the clock every day to figure out when to guzzle the next protein shake or have our mid-morning snack. If we don't our gym efforts will go to waste, right?

The idea of reducing our protein intake – even on the advice of hugely respected experts like Dr Ellington Darden – terrifies most weightlifters (aka protein addicts) like you and me. Let's look at some of the main reasons why:

#1 The Fear That Cutting Down On Protein Will Result In Muscle Loss

This is without doubt the biggest worry. The standard advice from the health and fitness industry is more protein = more muscle, and so we keep increasing it as we get bigger and stronger. Here are three examples that completely debunk this theory.

1 – Mike Mentzer was a bodybuilding champion who won the Mr Universe title in 1978 and in 1979 won the heavyweight class of the Mr Olympia competition...both with perfect 300 scores.

Mike's daily protein intake....60g per day. Yes, just 60g per day for a heavyweight competing athlete. Of course, genetics come into play but it still proves that we don't need to go overboard with protein. Mike placed more emphasis on calories than excessive protein intake.

Before he died in 2001, Mike said: *"Protein requirements depend almost entirely on your bodyweight, not your level of physical activity, because it is not used as fuel as long as the body's energy supply is adequate. The rule of thumb is one gram of protein per day for every two pounds of bodyweight."* Mike also insisted that buying expensive supplements was a waste of money because we can get what we need from a balanced diet which includes meat, fish or dairy products.

<u>2</u> – Dr Nick Delgado is a nutritional expert who tells us the same thing. He insists we require way less protein than we think – and also maintains that sufficient calories are more important. He follows a vegan diet and only eats around 60g of protein per day. In that case, you might imagine he's a bit of a weakling eh? Afraid not, Dr Delgado holds a world strength endurance record in the Guinness Book of Records for pressing the most weight overhead in an hour (53,640 pounds!) Dr Delgado says that it's important we take in enough calories, arguing that a protein intake of between 45g and 75g is generous.

<u>3</u> – I mentioned earlier that even Arnold Schwarzenegger consumed around 150g of protein per day (around 0.7g per 1lb of bodyweight). This is still relatively small for a 220lb guy who was training hard for the Mr Olympia world titles. Yet, I don't think anybody could argue with his results.

Also, a study was carried out in 2010 on 8 healthy men, who were each given infusions of amino acids (the building blocks of protein) over three hours. Protein synthesis increased with the influx of more amino acids – but then it began to decrease even though more amino acids were still being given. This suggests that bombarding the body with more protein does not necessarily mean more muscle.

#2 The Worry That It Will Lead To Too Much Weight Loss

Protein is not the body's primary fuel supply, carbohydrates are. By eating a sufficient amount of <u>complex</u> carbs and healthy fats too you can ensure the body's caloric needs are met. This helps maintain an ideal bodyweight, and has a protein sparing effect allowing you to develop muscle through strength training. For 'hard-gainers' like myself who struggle to add a pound of weight (but can easily lose two or three after a weekend on the booze), it is a good move to focus on increasing healthy fats. Fat contains 9 calories per gram, while protein and carbs contain just 4 grams each. On your shopping list add more nut butters, coconut milk, coconut oil, butter, olive oil, avocados etc.

#3 The Fear Of Gaining Too Much Weight

The complete opposite to the worry above, but a genuine fear for people who have slimmed down by following a high protein diet and by training hard. Our bodies are all different in terms of composition, metabolism, how well we process some foods etc. BUT – if you reduce your excessive protein intake and still stick to a diet that is largely made up of whole foods (i.e. plenty fresh veg and fruit, whole grains, no processed junk) then it's very difficult to go wrong...particularly if you're also lifting heavy.

The Protein Scale For A Weightlifter

Okay, so there are plenty of different opinions about how much protein we need to maintain and build muscle. And we obviously know this varies based on bodyweight. But let's look at the scale based on the information and the people referred to in this article.

- World Health Organisation – 35g.

- Dr Nick Delgado, world strength endurance champion - 45g-75g.

- Mike Mentzer, former Mr Universe and Mr Olympia - 1g of protein per 2lbs of bodyweight.

- Arnold Schwarzenegger - 1g of protein per 2.2lbs of bodyweight.

- Standard bodybuilding community recommendation – 1g of protein per 1lb of bodyweight.

- Advice from some protein supplement companies – 300g-400g per day.

Starting at the bottom end...let's be honest, you would probably eat that much before lunchtime. The World Health Organisation is also giving recommendations for the average person, not someone who lifts weight regularly. Going to the other end of the scale, these figures of 300g-400g are crazy, needless amounts. Dr Ellington Darden's detailed two-month long study clearly showed that large amounts of protein goes to waste.

The standard bodybuilding advice is that we must eat 1g of protein per 1lb of bodyweight. This figure has been around for decades...yet we don't know who made it up and on what basis. Yet two of the finest bodybuilders the world has ever produced are telling us we only need HALF that amount. This advice from Arnie and Mike Mentzer lies slap bang in the middle of the scale and is what I would consider the most sensible.

My recommendation: **1g of protein per 2lbs of bodyweight** is an ideal target to aim for.....but, crucially, supported by a sufficient number of calories from complex carbohydrates and healthy fats.

CHECKLIST

- **Heavy weight training does NOT require a massive protein intake**

- **Protein absorption is key – and both digestive issues and different types of foods are factors in this.**

- **Eat 1g of protein per 2lbs of bodyweight.**

- **This should be backed up with sufficient calories, which are equally important in the muscle building process.**

- **Our bodies can recycle amino acids, meaning there is no need for eating sky high amounts of protein.**

Chapter 7:

Pre-Workout Nutrition

We all have the same gym pre-workout problem...

Trying to figure out exactly what the hell to eat/drink/gorge on for enough energy to get through a tough gym session and make the best gains possible. On one hand we want to feast on plenty of food for fuel. On the other we don't want it to leave us feeling like we need a nap afterwards!

"Load up on carbs for energy," they tell us. I tried the big plate of pasta mid-afternoon. Left me feeling like a balloon.

"Drink a meal replacement shake for extra calories," they said. Somehow that left me feeling like a human slug by the time I started lifting weights.

Or the plain old banana that everyone tells you is a great source of energy. They're clearly bending the truth with that one. And don't get me started on those rubbish energy drinks. They contain ridiculously high amounts of sugar, all sorts of chemicals and additives, and if you'd like another reason not to drink them then Google "energy drinks deaths". Fact is: nothing really cut it – until I came across The Two 'C's. One natural supplement. One drink you probably have every day. Both beginning with the letter 'C'.

The Two 'C's: Coffee and Creatine

A plain cuppa black <u>coffee</u> and some <u>creatine</u> = an outrageously good combo for firing up your energy levels and boosting your performance in the gym. Taking these on an empty stomach ahead of a morning workout is highly effective for burning fat. This also sets the body up to be in a highly anabolic state when you have your post-workout meal.

I first heard about creatine around 15 years ago when I was still at college. I was out drinking on a summer's night at a local pub and I spotted a guy who was in my year at school. I hadn't seen him for a couple of years and the first thing I noticed was how big his arms and shoulders were. He had morphed into this muscle mutha and it didn't look like he had been taking anything dodgy like steroids. He was just in much better shape compared to last time I'd seen him.

Must admit, I remember feeling pretty gutted in that moment. I had been training pretty hard for around three years at that point and saw *some* gains, but looking at this dude was like a slap in the face waking me up. I figured that either I wasn't training hard enough – or I had just been going the wrong way about my weight training completely. So I pulled him aside and – while trying not to sound like a jealous weirdo who had been eyeing up another guy's muscles at the pub – I asked: *"Mate, you're in great shape. You must be training constantly. What are you doing exactly?"*

It was then he told me he had been taking creatine as a pre-workout supplement, along with the same brand's protein powder post-workout....and had <u>gained about 10lbs of muscle in a matter of months</u>. It had always been a nightmare for me to gain just two or three pounds. So I was sold on this stuff already. The next day I headed to the shop in Glasgow where my ex schoolmate bought his creatine. The creatine worked a treat. I put on around 6 or 7 pounds within the first couple of months and my strength went through the roof. I go through cycles of taking creatine now (two months on, one month off), but still get the same boost in power and performance in the gym 15 years later.

Creatine – The What, Why And How

<u>Basic science behind creatine</u>: it's an amino acid that's found in various foods and is also naturally produced in the body, helping to deliver energy to all cells, primarily muscles. Creatine increases the formation of ATP (adenosine triphosphate), which is the molecule that fuels life. ATP is where our cells get the energy to perform tasks. Essentially, more creatine = more ATP = more energy and power for workouts.

<u>How it works</u>: creatine has been proven to be effective in improving performance in weightlifters and other athletes. This is because it increases the body's ability to produce more energy rapidly, meaning you can train harder and for longer.

<u>How to get more of it</u>: beef and salmon are among the best food sources of creatine – but you would have to eat silly amounts to get the levels you need. That's why, since 1993, creatine has become a popular supplement in powder/capsules for athletes. There are several forms of this supplement but creatine *monohydrate* has been shown to be the most effective and is the most widely used.

The Benefits Of Supplementing With Creatine

As well as leading to an <u>improvement in strength</u> and an <u>increased capacity for high intensity work</u>, supplementing with creatine can reap various other benefits including:

<u>Fuller muscles</u> – creatine enhances the volume of muscles. This is mainly achieved through increasing the fluid content of the muscles. It pulls more water in, giving them a fuller look.

<u>Enhanced recovery</u> – a study on creatine supplementation was carried out in 2004 involving 34 men running a 30km race. Eighteen men used 20g of creatine mixed with maltodextrine per day for five days, while the others used only maltodextrine. Closely monitoring several markers of cell damage in both groups, researchers concluded: *"Creatine supplementation reduced cell damage and inflammation after an exhaustive intense race."*

<u>Better brain function</u> – creatine supplementation can improve short term memory and also protect against neurological disorders, studies suggest. In 2003, a study was carried out on 45 young adults where they took 5g of creatine per day for six weeks, then took tests on memory performance and intelligence. Researchers concluded that *"creatine supplementation had a significant positive effect"*.

Is Supplementing With Creatine Safe?

First off, it's worth reminding that creatine is not a drug of any sort. It's a natural compound produced in the body and that can also be absorbed from various food sources. There have been scare stories over the years that prolonged use of creatine can cause kidney problems, but this has been disproven in countless studies. Other negative effects have also been highlighted, such as stomach cramps.

These supposed side effects are all well addressed in an article titled *'Six Side Effects Of Creatine: Myths Debunked'*, which was published on Bodybuilding.com in November 2015. This well-researched, in-depth report is definitely worth a read if you have any concerns about taking creatine for the first time. The article underlines why it's a safe and effective supplement for healthy individuals and is backed up by 31 different studies.

- NOTE: People diagnosed with gout are advised not to take creatine as it will worsen the condition. If you have any health issues at all consult your doctor first before taking creatine.

How much should I take – and what about the 'loading phase'?

Dr Richard Kreider Phd gave a formula for working out how much creatine to take at first and then for daily maintenance. Dr Kreider is professor and head of the Department of Health and Kinesiology at Texas A&M University. He has published more than 300 sports nutrition articles and abstracts in scientific journals.

He advises that we initially increase muscle creatine stores by taking 0.3g per kg of bodyweight per day. Take this amount for 5-7 days and then simply take 3g-5g per day to maintain creatine stores. So an 80kg guy would take 24-25g for the first week and then reduce it to 5g daily. Or a 65kg woman would take 20g for the first week and then cut down to between 3g and 5g per day.

Stir Up Your Training Performance With Coffee

A cuppa coffee – without the sugar and cream – is an excellent pre-workout drink. It is a much healthier, safer choice than energy drinks. A simple black coffee an hour before your workout can provide the following benefits:

Increased energy – the high caffeine levels in coffee can provide a perfect power-up shortly before you hit the gym.

More fat loss – coffee, when consumed before a workout, can cause fatty acids to be used for energy rather than glycogen. The caffeine content also speeds up metabolism, which means more fat is burned throughout the day.

Better performance – coffee can be the difference between squeezing out a few more reps in the gym, or shaving a few seconds off your running time.

This was proven back in 1992 when a group of athletes were given 3g of coffee before a 1500m treadmill run. The study, published in the British Journal of Sports Medicine, showed that those who drank the coffee finished their run 4.2 secs faster on average than the control group. Other research also points to coffee helping to improve focus, decrease muscle pain during your workouts and even having a positive effect on your memory. So, while coffee is often seen as a vice by some people, it can actually have a positive impact when it comes to your training. Black and organic is best, and it's best sticking with the following advice:

Don't go overboard. Health experts recommend that no more than 400mg of caffeine (roughly three mugs of coffee) is consumed per day, while the limit is half that amount for pregnant women. Side effects of excessive caffeine intake include an increased heart rate and insomnia. Coffee is also acidic and too much acidity in the body leads to inflammation. Chronic inflammation depresses the immune system and can lead to health problems. Stay balanced by including plenty of vegetables and fruits, and natural, whole foods.

<u>Choose freshly-made coffee</u> – made with organic coffee beans if possible. Quality coffee beans contain various nutrients and flavonoid antioxidants, which help maintain good health. The processing of roasted coffee granules robs coffee of these nutrients.

<u>Cut out the sugar and cream</u>. Unless your coffee is black you're defeating the purpose. Sugar will not only spike your insulin levels – and come crashing down later – but too much of the white stuff is also converted into fatty acids in the liver. Meaning more fat on your belly, legs, arms…or wherever else you don't want it.

CHECKLIST

- A great pre-workout combo is black coffee and creatine.

- The coffee will help boost energy and burn fat, and can have a positive impact on your performance in the gym.

- Creatine can help you gain muscle mass by enhancing your performance, strength, and your recovery after training. It can also give your muscles a fuller look by drawing more water into the muscles.

- Begin a creatine 'loading phase' of taking around 0.3g per kg of bodyweight for 5-7 days.

- Creatine supplementation thereafter should be reduced to 3g-5g per day.

- I take creatine in cycles, two months on and one month off. People with gout are advised not to take creatine as it will worsen the condition. If you have any health issues consult your doctor first.

- A coffee (no sugar or cream) an hour before your workout can increase energy levels, boost performance and burn fat more efficiently.

- Due to its high caffeine content, you should drink no more than 3 mugs of coffee per day.

- Choose freshly ground organic brand of coffee rather than instant, which has been stripped of its antioxidants and isn't as effective.

Chapter 8:

Post-Workout Nutrition

When I first started out lifting weights when I was aged 16 I didn't have a clue about what I should be eating to try and build muscle. I can remember my friend Bryan and I training with a weight bench in his gran's house. Within seconds of finishing our last rep we were drinking pints of milk and wolfing down slice after slice of wafer thin honey roast ham. Wasn't exactly the tastiest combo but I'd read somewhere that milk helps you build muscle. These days I don't drink the stuff at all, but it's important to underline that it's not just what you eat, but when too.

The <u>two hour period</u> following your workout is prime time for making the most of your gym efforts. Ori Hofmekler, world leading sports nutritionist and author, describes it as the 'window of opportunity' for maximising muscle growth. Your body will temporarily be in a catabolic (muscle wasting) state following each weight training session. This is because the strain of intense exercise triggers the release of stress hormone cortisol in the body, which breaks down muscle tissue.

Doesn't sound good, right? But this biological process actually sets you up for flipping it into an anabolic (muscle building) state through proper nutrition afterwards. By flooding your body with the right nutrients – within the right timeframe – you halt the catabolic process and kickstart some serious muscle building as your body begins the growth and recovery phase following tough work done in the gym.

Feed Your Hungry Muscles Twice Within The Window Of Opportunity

The sooner we switch from catabolic to anabolic the better for muscle growth. This is where two post-workout 'feeds' come into play.

'Feed' 1

<u>Within 30 mins of your workout</u>: feed your muscles with fast assimilating protein to start the muscle building process. I recommend a plant-based protein shake, such as brown rice or vegan blend protein powder. Mixed with water, these are really easy for the body to absorb without any digestive issues.

'Feed' 2

<u>60-90 minutes later</u>: eat a healthy meal with a good balance of protein, complex carbs and healthy fats. These should come from the food sources mentioned in chapter 4. Not a good cook? There are tons of excellent cook books out there.

I recently pulled together all my favourite clean eating recipes and published *'Meal Prep Recipe Book: 50 Simple Recipes For Health & Fitness Nuts'*. The recipes are so tasty and the majority of them are ready in less than 30 minutes. To make life even easier, I also provide a breakdown of calories, protein, carbs and fats for each meal. Meal Prep Recipe Book is the next title in this two books combo.

CHECKLIST

- The <u>two hour period</u> following your workout is prime time for making the most of your gym efforts.

- Aim for two 'feeds' (which is really just a shake and one meal) in this 'window of opportunity' for maximising muscle growth.

- I recommend a plant-based protein powder shake with water 30 minutes after finishing your workout.

- Then 60-90 minutes after your shake have a nutritious meal composed of good sources of protein, complex carbs and healthy fats as described in chapter 4.

Chapter 9

Supplements: The Good, The Bad & The Useless

There's bodybuilding. And there's building a strong, healthy body. I class the two completely differently. I'd never consider myself a bodybuilder. A meathead bodybuilder probably wouldn't consider me a bodybuilder either. I'm cool with that. I'm just a guy who lifts heavy weights - and my health is of the utmost importance.

In my experience, I've seen too many bodybuilders put aesthetics, competition and their egos before their health. Just to get ahead, to try and be bigger or better than others, while not really thinking about any long-term consequences. Firstly, anyone who even considers taking steroids for a better body is not only a meathead, but a plain moron. You become fake, a fraud...and I won't bore you with the ball-shrinkingly frightening health dangers.

Secondly, anyone who takes other unnatural, synthetic pills, powders or liquids without properly doing their homework should also receive a 'moron' tattoo along with their gym membership.

"Take care of your body, it's the only place you have to live." – *Jim Rohn.*

Truth is: you don't need to waste your money on a bunch of supplements, dodgy or otherwise, to achieve the great body you want. A clean, healthy whole foods diet can provide virtually all you need. Having said that, there are still a handful of natural supplements that'll help you get the job done much more efficiently and effectively. I'll detail the 'essentials' and 'extras' I use to supplement my weight training program - and properly look after my body. They're safe, natural and opting for these will not only bring you excellent results, but it'll save you time, experimenting with garbage products, and a heck of a lot of money.

In part two of this chapter we'll also cover pre-workout and post-workout nutrition, which can be a headache for even the most experienced weightlifter. I'll share my 'ultimate pre-workout combo' for peak performance in the gym, aswell as tips on what to consume afterwards to gain the most from your monster gym efforts.

'The Essentials' – stock up on these whenever you get the chance

Multi-vitamin and mineral tablet

The body uses vitamins and minerals to repair and replace cells. We simply cannot function without these nutrients. The standard Western diet and the processing of food strips what we eat of its goodness. The result? Vitamin and mineral deficiencies. These deficiencies lead to various health problems. For example, if you lack vitamin B12 you'll likely feel tired, out of breath, or develop headaches.

It's like a car that needs oil and the warning light comes on. The body gives us plenty of warning signs too and it's up to us to give the body what it needs before it breaks down. But even eating plenty of organic fruit and veg isn't necessarily enough to cover all vitamin and mineral bases. So buying a good multivitamin and mineral supplement is a wise investment for foundational health.

Creatine

This could well be your weightlifting best friend. As described earlier, creatine has been proven to be effective in improving performance in weightlifters and other athletes. It increases the body's ability to produce energy more rapidly, meaning you can train harder – and for longer. Did I mention the benefits of fuller muscles, or enhanced recovery after workouts too? Creatine is an amino acid that's found in various foods and is naturally produced by the body too.

Plant-based protein powder

No I'm NOT talking about whey isolate protein powder. I ain't a fan of the usual type of protein that 98% of weightlifters/athletes/gym-goers drink to help build muscle. In my experience, many (not all) brands of whey protein are highly processed, contain chemicals and additives, and are acidic which makes it harder to digest and it has been argued that they can damage your health in the long term.

Myself and several friends suffered digestive problems after years of guzzling whey protein shakes. When we switched to an organic plant-based protein powder all the issues stopped. You only have to jump onto weight training and bodybuilding online forums to read countless complaints from people about how they feel sick, bloated and have toxic farts after drinking their protein shakes. Plant-based protein powders are much more alkaline and easily absorbed by the body. My advice is to ditch whey protein, buy the plant-based stuff instead.

Magnesium oil

Magnesium plays so many roles in the healthy functioning of our bodies, and is crucial for sports performance and recovery. But this mineral is also very easily depleted in our fast-paced, stressful lives. Intense exercise, such as heavy weight training can also further lower levels of magnesium and therefore it's a very wise move to supplement with magnesium oil. Dr Mark Sircus, author of Transdermal Magnesium Therapy, refers to magnesium as "by far the most important mineral in the body".

When it comes to performance: the body's main energy source ATP (adenosine triphosphate) must be bound to a magnesium ion in order to be biologically active. A deficiency in magnesium can therefore impair athletic performance. When it comes to recovery: supplementing with magnesium oil is hugely beneficial for people lifting weights because it relaxes and soothes sore muscles, speeding up recovery times after tough workouts.

It's also an amazing aid for a deep, restful sleep as it calms the nervous system by inhibiting the major stress hormones cortisol and adrenaline. Proper sleep is extremely important for muscle development and overall health. Spraying magnesium chloride oil on to the skin has been shown to be most effective for absorption.

'The Extras' – beneficial but not completely necessary if you don't have the cash

ZMA (Zinc, Magnesium, Vitamin B6)

This combination of two minerals and one vitamin is a potent mix for recovery and growth because it assists in achieving deep levels of sleep and hormone production. Training hard in the gym consistently can lower levels of testosterone, as can the stresses of everyday life. ZMA has been clinically proven to increase anabolic hormone levels and muscle strength in athletes. Studies have shown that it can increase the testosterone levels of men by around one third.

Greens powder

We all know how good vegetables are for us. But let's be honest, most of us don't eat anywhere near enough of them. Even those who do eat plenty are probably not getting enough nutrients from them because over-cooking strips vegetables of vitamins, minerals and natural enzymes. This is where a greens powder supplement can make all the difference. Packed with antioxidants and phytonutrients, this supplement is powerful for cleansing the entire body and protecting your cells. This can boost your immune system, improve digestion, and support overall health and wellbeing.

Digestive enzymes

Enzymes are produced by the body to break down our food properly and absorb the nutrients. They're also found in whole unprocessed foods such as fruit and veg. There are two problems: first, the body can struggle when faced with a constant influx of processed junk food and large volumes of animal protein, as found in the typical Western diet.

Heartburn, bloating, too much gas etc are all signs the body is having a hard time digesting what's been eaten. Secondly, cooking also robs foods of their natural enzymes. Digestive enzyme supplements can assist the body in breaking down larger volumes of food, such as cooked main meals. This means you get more out of what you eat, which of course provides the nutrients needed for muscle growth - and optimal health.

I've created a special supplements guide as a bonus for all readers of this book. The report lists my favourite supplements brands and how and when to take them. You can download it for free on my website at: www.weighttrainingistheway.com/supplements-guide

CHECKLIST

- The 'essentials' supplements are: multivitamin and mineral tablets, creatine, plant-based protein powder and magnesium oil.

- Multivitamins and minerals: these are important for addressing nutritional deficiencies that are common in the typical western diet and building good foundational health.

- Protein powder: choose an organic plant-based option, such as brown rice or vegan blend, over whey isolate protein. Not only because it is a highly absorbable form of protein, but because it's alkaline and therefore kinder to your insides than other highly processed, acidic brands.

- Magnesium oil: the huge role magnesium plays in sports performance, recovery and overall health is not widely known. It's also very easily depleted, especially following intense training. Stay one step ahead and look after your body well by supplementing with this magic mineral.

- The 'extras' supplements – if you've got the cash – are: ZMA capsules, greens powder and digestive enzymes.

Conclusion

I don't think anything I've explained in this book is hard to understand or follow. That's exactly the point. Proper nutrition / a clean diet / a healthy way of eating...whatever you want to call it...should be straightforward and easy to maintain. I take the same approach with my strength training programs too. Otherwise, we end up in a never ending cycle of becoming temporarily enslaved to a fad diet >> making progress >> inevitably having a major blowout >> losing our way and feeling like crap >> beating ourselves up >> and then it's back to square one.

Does it not make more sense to just get all the basics right consistently? You know, like...

- Cutting down on sugar

- Limiting the booze

- Eating more vegetables and fruit

- Keeping an eye on your calories

- Drinking plenty of water and taking a vitamin and mineral supplement every day

Doing all of the above isn't hard work. Making good food choices – as described in chapter 4 – Monday-Friday ain't that difficult either. Especially when you can relax a bit and enjoy treats at the weekend. None of that sounds like a diet to me. It's simply a healthy eating lifestyle and will provide your body with what it needs as you progress on your strength training program.

As for training itself, I've experimented with all sorts of foods, drinks and supplements to give me fuel and boost my performance in the gym. Forget all these dodgy energy drinks or hyped-up supplements, a black coffee and creatine is the way forward. My energy and strength levels go through the roof with this combo. If you're overweight then I'd go only with the coffee and leave out the creatine until you're close to your target weight. This is because creatine pulls water into your muscles and water retention isn't what you want.

As for the coffee, make sure it's black and go for a freshly made organic brew instead of instant. Remember to fully capitalise on your gym efforts by having two post-workout feeds within the two hour 'window of opportunity'. I have my plant-based protein powder shake 30 minutes after finishing my workout, and then follow this up around 60 minutes later with a nutritious meal such as oatcakes and tuna mayonnaise, or one of my special calorific super shakes!

You don't necessarily need to blow your cash on supplements to help you build muscle, strip fat and get in better overall shape. But, as I mentioned in the last chapter, there are some essentials and non-essentials which I use to complement my training regime and optimise my health. They're all completely natural, fairly cheap, and are worth every penny.

My special supplements guide is available as a bonus for all readers of this book. The report lists my favourite supplement brands and how and when to take them. You can download it for free on my website by visiting:
www.weighttrainingistheway.com/supplements-guide

I Forgot....

I hope you've enjoyed reading this book and it helps you become a stronger, better, healthier version of yourself. If you have any questions about anything in the book feel free to email me at: marc@weighttrainingistheway.com

I'd be massively, ridiculously grateful if you went over to Amazon and left me a review of this book. Right, enough reading. Get back to the gym!

All the best, Marc McLean.

Bibliography / Further Reading / References

Essentials of Strength Training and Conditioning, 3rd edition – Baechle, Earle.

The Warrior Diet – Ori Hofmekler.

Eat Stop Eat – Brad Pilon.

Paul M La Bounty, Bill I Campbell, Jacob Wilson, Elfego Galvan, John Berardi,

Susan M Kleiner, Richard B Kreider,
Jeffrey R Stout,Tim Ziegenfuss, Marie Spano, Abbie Smith and Jose Antonio. March 2011. International Society of Sports Nutrition position stand: meal frequency. http://www.jissn.com/content/8/1/4

MM Manore. August 2005. Exercise and the Institute of Medicine recommendations for nutrition.
http://www.ncbi.nlm.nih.gov/pubmed/16004827

R Estruch, E Ros, J Salas-Salvado, M Isabel-Covas, D Pharm, D Corella, F Aros, E Gomez-Gracia, V Ruiz-Gutierrez, M Fiol, J Lapetra, RM Lamuela-Raventos, L Serra Majem, X Pinto, J Pasora, M A Munoz, J V Sorli, J A Martinez, M A Martinez-Gonzalez. Primary Prevention of Cardiovascular Disease with a Mediterranean Diet. April 2013.
http://www.nejm.org/doi/full/10.1056/NEJMoa1200303

P J Atherton, T Etheridge, P W Watt, D Wilkinson, A Selby, D Rankin, K Smith, M J Rennie. November 2010. Muscle full effect after oral protein: time-dependent concordance and discordance between human muscle protein synthesis and mTORC1 signaling.
http://www.ncbi.nlm.nih.gov/pubmed/20844073

J D Wiles, S R Bird, J Hopkins and M Riley. June 1992. Effect of caffeinated coffee on running speed, respiratory factors, blood lactate and perceived exertion during 1500-m treadmill running.

British Journal of Sports Medicine. https://www.ncbi.nlm.nih.gov/pmc/articles/PMC1478936/

C Rae, A L Digney, S R McEwan, T C Bates. October 2003. Oral creatine monohydrate supplementation improves brain performance: a double-blind, placebo-controlled, cross-over trial. https://www.ncbi.nlm.nih.gov/pubmed/14561278

R V Santos, R A Bassit, E C Caperuto, L F Costa Rosa. September 2004. The effect of creatine supplementation upon inflammatory and muscle soreness markers after a 30km race.

https://www.ncbi.nlm.nih.gov/pubmed/15306159

Meal Prep:

50 Simple Recipes For Health & Fitness Nuts

Introduction

Cooking can be a pain in the @ss sometimes...

But so is the struggle to shift stubborn flab around your belly, or gain lean muscle, if you're not eating the right foods every day.

Your exercise efforts will go to waste if you don't back them up with good sources of protein, carbs and fats, and sufficient calories for your health and fitness goals.

No need to worry about that...because this book serves up 50 awesome recipes that are simple to make - and ridiculously tasty. These nutrient-packed recipes make clean eating easy and prove that you don't have to eat boring, bland food to get in great shape.

Each recipe also includes a calorie and macronutrients breakdown. Keeping track of calories, carbs or grams of protein couldn't be easier.

Ready meals, takeaways, and most foods that come pre-packaged from the supermarket shelves don't do us any good. Processed to the point where they become 'dead foods' – i.e. most of the nutritional value has been stripped away, or they have been loaded with sugar, salt, additives and chemicals.

The answer – cook using fresh ingredients. Then you know exactly what is going into your meal and can take full charge of your daily nutrition.

I also want my meals to be as quick and easy as possible because...I'll be honest...I'm hardly a masterchef. But you don't have to be either to be able to prepare and produce tasty, healthy, fresh food.

I was never looking for Michelin star type meals, I just wanted recipes that ticked three boxes....

- Healthy
- Tasty
- Pretty easy to cook

After years of stuffing my face with some awesome grub, I've pulled together my best of the bunch. These include:

- 10 main meals (all ridiculously tasty)
- 10 breakfasts (with plenty of variety)
- 10 soup recipes (simple and delicious)
- 10 'power shake' recipes (jam-packed with vitamins and minerals)
- 10 healthy snacks (sooo good you wouldn't believe they're healthy)

Some recipes are very basic. Some are a *little bit* more fancy...but you still won't find it difficult to cook them. Finally, the majority of recipes take less than 30 mins to prepare.

These are my personal favourite recipes...the ones I keep going back to. They're ideal for people who lift weights like me, or exercise regularly and are looking for nutritious food to not only fuel their workouts, but help their body recover and develop afterwards.

I share these recipes with my online personal training clients who love most of them. (The sweet potato and chickpea curry main meal, and mango power shake, are among the favourites!) Freshly cooked meals will help keep your waistline trim and help you sculpt a strong, athletic, awesome physique.

Enjoy!

Marc McLean

Online Personal Training & Nutrition Coach // Health & Fitness author // Food Lover

www.weighttrainingistheway.com

Breakfasts

Berry Crunch

Spiced-Up Scrambled Eggs

Creamy leeks and Eggs

Peanut Butter & Banana Porridge

Hot Fruit & Nuts Cereal

Fruity Oats

Protein Pancakes

Broccoli Bake

Pepper & Onion Omelette

Quinoa Fruit Salad

Main Meals

Turkey Chilli

Sweet Potato & Chickpea Curry

Paella Power

Creamy Garlic Pasta

Salmon & Veg Special

Chicken, Broccoli & Spinach Pie

Piri Piri Chicken

Veggie Chilli

Chicken Thighs With Sweet Potato

Chicken Satay Supreme

Soup-er Soups

Spiced Lentil & Veg

Chicken & Rice

Sweet Potato & Pepper

Leek & Potato

Pea, Leek & Bacon

Creamy Carrot & Parsnip

Salmon & Veg

Creamy Chicken, Potato & Bacon

Mixed Bean

Split Pea & Courgette

Healthy Snacks

Nut Protein Bars

Coconut Protein Balls

Simple Protein Cookies

Sweet As A Nut Balls

Choc Coconut Cookie Balls

No Bake Brilliant Bars

Cranberry Coconut Balls

Delicious Dates Bites

Protein Raisin Cookies

Almond Fudge Bars

Power Shakes

Blueberry Blast

Choc n' Banana

Mango Monster

Avocado Attack

Strawberry Goji Smooth

Tropical Twist

Green Pineapple Power

Ginger Booster

Chia Berry

Tropical Treat

Berry Crunch

Ingredients

1 cup natural Greek Yoghurt

1/4 cup blueberries

1/2 sliced banana

Handful of almonds

1/4 cup granola (aim for less than 20g of sugar per 100g)

Sprinkle of cinnamon

1 tsp of honey

Servings - 1

Nutrition per serving

Calories: 449

Protein: 31g

Carbs: 58g

Fat: 31g

Step 1

Pour the cup of natural Greek yoghurt into a bowl.

Step 2

Add the granola, banana slices, almonds, and blueberries.

Step 3

Sprinkle over the cinnamon and drizzle with honey.

Spiced-up Scrambled Eggs

Ingredients   **Servings - 1**

3 slices of thin chorizo slices/pepperoni slices   **Nutrition   per serving**

3 eggs

2.5 tbsp butter   Calories: 712

2 slices wholemeal bread   Protein: 37g

1/2 white onion   Carbs: 36g

Roughly 1 tbsp grated cheddar cheese   Fat: 44g

Sea salt and pepper

Step 1

Put 1.5 tbsp of butter in a saucepan over a low to medium low heat, dice the onion and then cook it in the butter until soft.

Step 2

While the onion is cooking, cut the chorizo/pepperoni slices into small pieces and then add to the saucepan.

Step 3

Mix up the eggs in a bowl with 1/2 tsp of salt and just a small dash of pepper.

Step 4

Pour eggs into the saucepan, add grated cheese, and continue to cook on a low to low medium heat until ready.

Step 5

Serve with wholemeal toast.

Creamy Leeks & Eggs

Ingredients

Servings - 2

4 leeks, chopped

Nutrition per serving

3 tbsp butter

3 tbsp single cream

Calories: 364

3 slices of crispy bacon Protein: 21g

5 eggs

Carbs: 28g

Fat: 18g

Step 1

Trim the leeks and chop them into small square pieces.

Step 2

Add 2 tbsp of butter to a saucepan and melt over a low heat.

Step 3

Add the leeks to the saucepan and cook for 5-6 mins until softened.

Step 4

Whisk 1 tbsp of single cream in a bowl together with the eggs, then season with salt and pepper.

Step 5

Melt the other tbsp of butter in another saucepan on a low heat, and then cook the eggs in it. Meanwhile, grill the bacon slices until they become crispy.

Step 6

Keep stirring the eggs so they don't become too firm. When the eggs are cooked, but still a little soft, divide them onto two plates.

Step 7

Add the other 2 tbsp of cream to the leeks and stir through.

Step 8

Top the eggs with the creamy leek mixture, then crumble the crispy bacon over the top.

Peanut & Banana Porridge

Ingredients

1/2 ripe banana

1 cup oats

1 cup almond milk or rice milk

1 tbsp natural unsweetened peanut butter

1 tsp honey

Servings - 1

Nutrition per serving

Calories: 507

Protein: 17g

Carbs: 79g

Fat: 16g

Step 1

Add the oats and almond milk to a saucepan and cook until the oats are softened and ready, adding more almond milk if necessary.

Step 2

Transfer the porridge oats to a large bowl and then slice up the half banana.

Step 3

Add the banana slices to the porridge, along with the tablespoon of peanut butter, and mix well.

Step 4

Drizzle a teaspoon of honey over the peanut and banana porridge mixture.

Hot Fruit & Nuts Cereal

Ingredients   **Servings - 2**

1/2 cup almonds   **Nutrition per serving**

1/2 cup cashews

1/2 ripe banana   Calories: 260

1/2 tsp of ground cinnamon   Protein: 9g

Pinch of salt   Carbs: 10g

100ml coconut milk   Fat: 22g

1 egg

Step 1

Add all ingredients to a blender or food processor and blitz until smooth.

Step 2

Warm the mixture on a medium heat for 5 mins.

Step

Serve and add almond milk, or some fresh berries, to suit your taste.

Fruity Oats

Ingredients

1 chopped pear

1/2 chopped apple

1 tbsp linseed

Handful of almonds

A splash of almond milk

1/2 cup oats

1 tsp honey

Servings - 1

Nutrition per serving

Calories: 454

Protein: 10g

Carbs: 73g

Fat: 11g

Step 1

Cook the oats as per instructions

Step 2

Meanwhile, chop the pear and apple into small chunks and place in a breakfast bowl, along with 6-8 almonds.

Step 3

Sprinkle the linseed over the fruit and pour over a little almond milk to moisten it.

Step 4

Pour the cooked oats over the fruit and nuts, then drizzle with honey and serve.

Protein Pancakes

Ingredients

3 medium free range eggs

1/2 cup oats

1 ripe banana

1 tbsp unsweetened peanut butter

1 tsp cinnamon

1-2 tsp honey

Servings - 3 pancakes

Nutrition per pancake

Calories: 229

Protein: 13g

Carbs: 36g

Fat: 12g

Step 1

Put the eggs, oats, peanut butter, banana and cinnamon into a blender and mix into a batter consistency

(Add a bit more oats if it's too runny).

Step 2

Put a frying pan on at low to medium heat and pour the mixture in to cook pancakes.

Step 3

Drizzle the pancakes with honey and serve.

Broccoli Bake

Ingredients

8 broccoli florets

6 eggs

1 can / 400ml coconut milk

1 tbsp butter

1/2 cup grated cheddar cheese

1/4 tsp nutmeg

Salt and pepper

Servings - 4

Nutrition per serving

Calories: 347

Protein: 13g

Carbs: 5g

Fat: 31g

Step 1

Preheat the oven to 200°C/400°F/gas 6

Step 2

Cook the broccoli in boiling water for 5 mins until nearly softened.

Step 3

Butter a 10 inch round or small baking dish.

Step 4

In a large mixing bowl, whisk together the eggs, coconut milk, butter, nutmeg, salt and pepper.

Step 5

Drain the broccoli and stir into the mixing bowl, along with the grated cheese.

Step 6

Pour the mixture into the baking dish and cook for 20 minutes.

Pepper & Onion Omelette

Ingredients

3 eggs

1 red pepper, diced

1/2 white onion, diced

50g feta cheese, crumbled

1 tbsp extra virgin olive oil

Sea salt and pepper

Servings - 1

Nutrition per serving

Calories: 532

Protein: 31g

Carbs: 15g

Fat: 39g

Step 1

Add 1 tbsp of extra virgin olive oil to a frying pan at a low-medium heat.

Step 2

Add the diced pepper pan and cook for a few minutes, then add the onion and continue cooking until both are soft.

Step 3

Whisk the eggs in a bowl and season with salt and pepper to taste.

Step 4

Pour the eggs into the pan and cook on the low-medium heat for 2-3 mins.

Step 5

Crumble the feta cheese over the top of the eggs in the pan. Then put the pan under the grill until the eggs are cooked on top (be careful not to leave it under for too long and overcook them).

Quinoa Fruit Salad

Ingredients   Servings - 4

1 cup quinoa   **Nutrition per serving**

1 cup strawberries, sliced

1 cup blueberries, sliced   Calories: 272

1 cup mango, diced   Protein: 6g

1 tbsp honey   Carbs: 60g

1 lime   Fat: 3g

1 tbsp of chopped fresh basil

Step 1

Cook the quinoa as per instructions on the packet and then leave to cool for 10-15 mins.

Step 2

Mix the quinoa in a large bowl along with the sliced and diced fruit.

Step 3

Squeeze the juice of the lime into a small bowl and mix with the honey.

Step 4

Drizzle the lime and honey mixture over the quinoa and fruit. Garnish with the chopped basil.

Main Meals

- **Most meal recipes provide 4 servings.**
- **Why not make a batch at night and take another serving into work for lunch the next day?**
- **If there's the odd ingredient you don't like feel free to swap them to suit your tastes.**

Turkey Chilli

Ingredients

1 tbsp extra virgin olive oil

500g lean ground turkey mince

1 red onion, chopped

1 red pepper, chopped

1 green pepper

4 cloves garlic, minced

2 green chilies, diced

1 tsp of chilli powder

1 can red kidney beans

1 packet chilli seasoning mix

1 cup of water

Sea salt and pepper.

Servings - 4

Nutrition per serving

Calories: 376

Protein: 40g

Carbs: 24g

Fat: 13g

Step 1

Add the extra virgin olive oil to a large saucepan and heat at medium.

Step 2

Add lean ground turkey mince cook until brown on both sides.

Step 3

Add all the remaining ingredients and keep stirring regularly for 5-10 mins.

Step 4

Season with salt and pepper, then turn the heat up and bring the chilli to a boil.

Step 5

Cover the chilli with a lid, turn the heat down to low and simmer for 30 mins before serving.

Sweet Potato & Chickpea Curry

Ingredients

1 tbsp coconut oil

1 red onion, diced

1 red chilli, de-seeded and chopped

2 cloves garlic, minced

1 tsp ground ginger

1 tsp turmeric powder

1 tsp chilli flakes

1 tsp chilli powder

1/2 tsp cumin

1/2 tsp ground coriander

200g white rice

400g chopped tomatoes

400g chickpeas

400ml coconut milk

2 medium sweet potatoes, peeled and chopped

Sea salt and pepper

1 bunch fresh coriander

1 lime

230ml coconut yoghurt

Servings - 4

Nutrition per serving

Calories: 605

Protein: 14g

Carbs: 54g

Fat: 35g

Step 1

Cut the sweet potatoes into small chunks and cook in boiling water for 15 mins until softened.

Step 2

While the potatoes are cooking, heat the coconut oil in a large pan or wok, then add the onion and cook for a few minutes until softened. Add the garlic, chilli, ginger and spices, along with salt and pepper, then stir well and fry gently for a further couple of minutes.

Step 3

Add in the tomatoes, chickpeas and coconut milk. Stir and turn the curry down to a simmer. Finely chop a small handful of the coriander stems, then stir those in too, before adding the juice of half a lime.

Step 4

Cook the white rice or quinoa as per instructions on the packet.

Step 5

Add the sweet potatoes to the curry mix in the large pan. Cover with a lid for around 20 mins, stirring a couple of times and adding more seasoning and spices depending on your taste.

Step 6

Just before you're ready to serve, stir through the coconut yoghurt, along with more lime and spices if desired. Serve with the boiled rice or quinoa.

Paella Power

Ingredients

500g chicken breast

500g prawns

1 tbsp extra virgin olive oil

3 cups short grain brown rice

400ml chicken stock

1/2 red onion

2 tomatoes

200g frozen peas

4 cloves garlic, minced

1 tablespoon of smoked paprika

Sea salt and pepper

Servings - 6

Nutrition per serving

Calories: 405

Protein: 42g

Carbs: 45g

Fat: 8g

Step 1

Cook rice according to the instructions on the packet and set aside.

Step 2

Chop chicken breasts into small chunks.

Step 3

Add the extra virgin olive oil to a wok or large skillet and warm up at a low-medium heat. Add the red onion and minced garlic, and cook until softened.

Step 4

Add in the chicken chunks, turn the cooker up to medium, and heat until the chicken is almost cooked through.

Step 5

Stir in the prawns and continue cooking for another 10 minutes.

Step 6

Add the paprika and sea salt and pepper to season. Stir well.

Step 7

Mix in the cooked rice, diced tomatoes, and keep stirring occasionally.

Step 8

Pour in the chicken stock and stir through.

Step 9

Add frozen peas in last and stir. Allow the paella to simmer for 5-10 minutes before serving.

Creamy Garlic Pasta

Ingredients

250g wholewheat penne pasta

400g cherry tomatoes, halved

2 medium shallots, sliced

8 garlic cloves, minced

2 tbsp extra virgin olive oil

4 tbsp of plain flour

400ml of almond milk

250ml of vegetable stock

Sea salt and pepper

Handful of fresh basil

Servings - 3

Nutrition per serving

Calories: 280

Protein: 6g

Carbs: 32g

Fat: 12g

Step 1

Preheat oven to 200°C/400°F/gas 6. Put the halved cherry tomatoes in a bowl and mix with the extra virgin olive oil and sea salt.

Step 2

Place the tomatoes (cut side up) in a baking tray and cook in the oven for 20 mins.

Step 3

Add boiling water to a large saucepan and cook the penne pasta according the instructions on the packet. Drain afterwards, cover and then set aside.

Step 4

In the meantime, add 1 tbsp of olive oil to a saucepan over a low-medium heat and then cook the garlic and shallots for a few minutes until softened. Season with salt and pepper.

Step 5

Stir in the flour and mix with a whisk. Slowly whisk in the almond milk a bit at a time so that clumps don't form. Then add in the vegetable stock.

Step 6

Add more salt and black pepper, turn up to a medium heat, and continue cooking for another 4-5 minutes to thicken.

Step 7

Keep stirring until the sauce reaches your desired thickness, then taste and add more salt and pepper if needed

Step 8

Add the pasta and roasted tomatoes and stir. Garnish with fresh basil.

Salmon & Veg Special

Ingredients

4 fresh skinless salmon fillets

2 large eggs

1 red onion, diced

2 garlic cloves, minced

3 tbsp extra virgin olive oil

2 tbsp red wine vinegar

200g asparagus, trimmed

100g garden peas

1 tsp finely chopped parsley

Sea salt and pepper

Servings - 4

Nutrition per serving

Calories: 437

Protein: 43g

Carbs: 3g

Fat: 26g

Step 1

Lightly grease kitchen foil on a baking tray and then place the salmon fillets on it.

Step 2

Season the salmon with salt and pepper before cooking in the oven at 180 degrees C / gas mark 4 for 12-15 mins.

Step 3

While the salmon is cooking, boil the eggs in a small saucepan. Then cool the eggs with cold water before cutting them into small, crumbly pieces.

Step 4

To make the vinaigrette, whisk together the diced red onion, red wine vinegar, olive oil and minced garlic in a mixing bowl. Season with salt and pepper.

Step 5

Bring a saucepan of salted water to the boil and cook the asparagus for 1 minute. Remove the asparagus, rinse with cold water and add to the vinaigrette, along with the garden peas.

Step 6

Sprinkle the chopped parsley into the vinaigrette bowl and toss the mixture.

Step 7

Place the salmon on plates, top with the vegetable mixture, and sprinkle the crumbled eggs over the top.

Chicken, Broccoli & Spinach Pie

Ingredients

2 skinless chicken breasts

6 broccoli florets

200g baby mushrooms, sliced

1/2 tsp of chilli flakes

Zest of 1 lemon

100g of spinach

8 sheets filo pastry

1 egg

25g butter

2 tbsp olive oil

Sea salt and pepper

Servings - 4

Nutrition per serving

Calories: 443

Protein: 26g

Carbs: 50g

Fat: 15g

Step 1

Preheat the oven to 180 degrees C / 350 degrees F. Place the chicken in a roasting tin, drizzled with 1 tbsp of olive oil and seasoned with salt and pepper. Cook for 20 mins until chicken is cooked through.

Step 2

While the chicken is in the oven, boil the broccoli in salted water for 10-15 mins until softened.

Step 3

Add 1 tbsp of extra virgin olive oil to a frying pan and cook the mushrooms on medium heat. Add the chilli flakes, lemon zest, and spinach and keep stirring until all the spinach is wilted.

Step 4

Stir the egg into the frying pan and season with salt and pepper.

Step 5

Cut the chicken into small chunks and add it to the spinach/mushroom mixture. Then mix in the broccoli.

Step 6

Brush a baking tin with butter and lay four sheets of filo pastry in the base to cover.

Step 7

Pour in half of the chicken and broccoli mixture, cover with two more filo pastry sheets, and then pour in the remaining chicken and broccoli mixture.

Step 8

Pull the sides of the pastry in, add the remaining sheets on top, and then tuck them down the sides of the pie.

Step 9

Brush the pastry with melted butter and mark the pastry into squares with a knife. Bake for 20 minutes 200°C/400°F/gas 6.

Piri Piri Chicken

Ingredients

4 chicken breasts

1 red pepper, sliced

1 yellow pepper, sliced

3 large sweet potatoes, diced

50g grated cheddar cheese

1-2 tsp ground oregano

6 sprigs of fresh thyme

1 red onion, diced

2 cloves garlic, minced

1 red chilli, diced

1 tbsp paprika

1 lemon

2 tbsp white wine vinegar

1 tbsp Worcestershire sauce

Sea salt and pepper

A bunch of fresh basil

Servings – 4

Nutrition per serving

Calories: 286

Protein: 26g

Carbs: 33g

Fat: 6g

Step 1

Slash the chicken breasts on each side a few times. Drizzle with olive oil, season with a little salt and pepper, and then cook in a griddle pan on a medium heat. Cook until golden underneath, then turn over.

Step 2

Peel and dice the sweet potatoes and boil in a saucepan of slightly salted water for 15 mins until softened.

Step 3

To make the piri piri sauce: add the red onion, garlic, chilli (stalks removed), paprika, the zest of 1 lemon and then its juice all together in a food processor. Add the white wine vinegar, Worcestershire sauce, bunch of basil, a couple of pinches of salt and pepper, along with a couple of splashes of water. Blend all ingredients until smooth.

Step 4

Add the sliced peppers to the pan alongside the chicken. Turn the heat down to low-medium and then turn the oven on to 200°C/400°F/gas 6.

Step 5

Pour the piri piri sauce into a casserole dish/roasting tray. Add the chicken and peppers to the tray next. Scatter over the sprigs of thyme, then put the tray into the middle of the oven.

Step 8

Drain the cooked potatoes and then mash them well in the saucepan, stir in the grated cheese, along with the oregano.

Step 9

Take the chicken out of the oven and check it's cooked through properly before serving alongside the potatoes.

Veggie Chilli

Ingredients

1 cup brown rice

400g pack of roasted vegetables

400g can of kidney beans, drained

400g can of chopped tomatoes

1 tsp medium chilli powder

1 tsp chilli flakes

1 green chilli, de-seeded and chopped

Sea salt and pepper

Servings - 2

Nutrition per serving

Calories: 472

Protein: 26g

Carbs: 80g

Fat: 10g

Step 1

Cook the rice in boiling water with some salt, according to instructions on packet.

Step 2

Preheat the oven to 200°C/400°F/gas 6. Cook the vegetables in baking tray for 15 mins until softened.

Step 3

Mixed in the kidney beans, chopped tomatoes, chilli powder, chilli flakes, and chopped green chilli. Stir through the vegetables and then season with some salt and pepper to suit your own tastes.

Step 4

Cook the veggie chilli mixture for another 10-15 mins in the oven.

Step 5

Drain rice and serve with the chilli.

Chicken Thighs With Sweet Potato

Ingredients

8 chicken thighs, skin on

1 tbsp mustard

1 tbsp honey

2 tbsp soy sauce

4 sweet potatoes, peeled and chopped

2 red peppers, chopped

1 tbsp extra virgin olive oil

Sea salt and pepper

100g baby spinach

Servings - 4

Nutrition per serving

Calories: 663

Protein: 42g

Carbs: 33g

Fat: 42g

Step 1

Preheat the oven to 200°C/400°F/gas 6. Boil the sweet potato slices in salted water for 5-6 mins until slightly softened then drain.

Step 2

Mix the mustard, honey and soy sauce together in a bowl, and season with salt and pepper.

Step 3

Mix the chicken thighs in the bowl until properly coated in the sauce.

Step 3

Heat the olive oil in a large frying pan over a medium heat. Cook the chicken, skin side down, in two batches for 4-5 mins until they start to brown. Turn over and cook the other side for 4-5 mins.

Step 4

Add the chicken to a roasting tin, along with the sweet potatoes and chopped peppers.

Step 5

Roast in the oven for 25 minutes until golden and the chicken is cooked through.

Step 6

Serve with washed baby spinach.

Chicken Satay Supreme

Ingredients

4 skinless chicken breasts

1 tsp of honey

1/2 small bunch of fresh coriander

1 fresh red chilli

1 clove of garlic, chopped

3 tbsp unsweetened peanut butter

2 tbsp soy sauce

1/2 tsp ground ginger

2 limes

(For the noodles)

250g thin egg noodles for pan frying

4 spring onions

2-3 cups bean sprouts

3 tbsp extra virgin olive oil

2 tbsp soy sauce

1 tsp brown sugar

Sea salt and pepper

Servings - 4

Nutrition per serving

Calories: 535

Protein: 54g

Carbs: 52g

Fat: 26g

Step 1

Turn the grill on to full and set out 4 metal skewers. (If you only have wooden ones soak them in water first).

Step 2

To make the satay sauce, put the following ingredients in a food processor: coriander, chilli (stalk removed), garlic, 3 tablespoons of peanut butter, 1/2 tsp of ginger, and a few splashes of soy sauce. Grate in the zest of both limes, then squeeze in the juice from 1 of them. Add a couple of splashes of water, a little salt and pepper, and then blend to a paste consistency.

Step 3

Spoon half of the satay sauce into a bowl, and the other half is to be used for the next step.

Step 4

Chop the 4 chicken breasts into small-medium sized chunks and then spear them with the skewers. Put them in a roasting tray and then use your hands to coat them well with half of the satay sauce.

Step 5

Drizzle the chicken with olive oil and season with sea salt. Put under the grill, for around 10 minutes on each side, or until golden and cooked through.

Step 6

While the chicken is cooking, rinse the spring onions and bean sprouts, and then chop the spring onions into small pieces. Put the noodles in a large bowl, cover with boiling water and a plate, then leave to soak for 2-3 minutes.

Step 7

Mix the soy sauces, sesame oil, sugar, salt and pepper in a small bowl and set aside. Put a wok over a medium-high heat with a tablespoon of oil to coat it.

Step 8

Spread the noodles evenly in the wok and tilt it in a circular motion to spread the oil.

Step 9

Turn the chicken skewers over to cook the other side then return to the wok and turn the noodles over too once they become crisp. Flip them over and add another tablespoon of oil around the wok to cook the other side.

Step 10

Add the chopped spring onions, beansprouts and sauce to the wok and toss continuously. Cook for no more than 1 minute so that the sprouts remain crunchy.

Step 12

Plate up the chicken and noodles and serve.

Soup-er Soups

- **Easy to make soups with plenty of vegetables.**
- **Ready in under an hour and the recipes provide 4 generous servings.**
- **Don't forget to season with salt and pepper to suit your own tastes.**

Spiced Lentil & Vegetable Soup

Ingredients

1 tbsp of extra virgin olive oil

1 tbsp of mild or medium curry powder

3 cloves of garlic, minced

2 litres of water

2 vegetable stock cubes

1 white onion, chopped

3 medium carrots, peeled and chopped

100g red lentils

1 parsnip, peeled and chopped

1 medium stalk of celery, chopped

1 tbsp of tomato puree

Sea salt and pepper

Servings - 4

Nutrition per serving

Calories: 115

Protein: 4g

Carbs: 20g

Fat: 3g

Step 1

Heat the oil in a soup pot, add the curry powder and garlic and stir over a low heat for 1 minute.

Step 2

Add the water, two stock cubes, and the rest of the ingredients and bring to the boil.

Step 3

Turn the heat down and season with salt and pepper. Put the lid on and cook for 35-40 mins.

Step 4

Puree with a hand blender, or using a food processor, and then serve.

Chicken & Rice Soup

Ingredients

2 chicken legs with skin on

2 medium carrots, peeled and grated

1 white onion, chopped

1/2 cup white rice

2 chicken stock cubes

2 litres of boiling water

Sea salt and pepper

Servings - 6

Nutrition per serving

Calories: 213

Protein: 9g

Carbs: 14g

Fat: 7g

Step 1

Pour the boiling water into the soup pot and dissolve the stock cubes.

Step 2

Add the chicken legs, then the rice and bring to the boil.

Step 3

Add in the grated carrots and chopped onion, and turn the heat down, allowing the pot to simmer for 30-40mins.

Step 4

Remove the chicken legs carefully and cut off all the remaining chicken from the bone. Then chuck this back into the pot.

Step 5

Season the soup with salt and pepper to suit your own tastes, then serve.

Sweet Potato & Pepper Soup

Ingredients

1 tsp of coconut oil

2 large sweet potatoes, peeled and chopped

2 red onions, chopped

1 red pepper, chopped

4 cloves of garlic, minced

2 litres of vegetable stock

Sea salt and pepper

Chopped parsley

Servings - 4

Nutrition per serving

Calories: 100

Protein: 2g

Carbs: 21g

Fat: 2g

Step 1

Heat the oil in a large pot and fry the onion and garlic for 3 minutes on low heat. Add in the sweet potato, carrot and bell pepper and cook for 5 minutes on high. Stir occasionally.

Step 2

Add the water and the vegetable stock cubes, bring to boil and simmer the soup for 20 minutes.

Step 3

Puree the soup with a hand blender, and season with salt and pepper.

Step 4

Garnish with a little chopped parsley and serve.

Leek & Potato Soup

Ingredients

2 tbsp butter

3 leeks, sliced

1 white onion, chopped

250g potatoes peeled and diced

850 ml of vegetable stock

150ml of single cream

Salt and pepper

Servings - 4

Nutrition per serving

Calories: 251

Protein: 4g

Carbs: 27g

Fat: 14g

Step 1

Prepare are the vegetables, slicing the leeks, chopping the onion, and then dicing the potatoes.

Step 2

Add the butter to a large saucepan and melt it over a low heat.

Step 3

Add the vegetables to the saucepan and saute for 3-4 mins until soft but not brown.

Step 4

Pour in the vegetable stock, increase the heat on the cooker and bring to the boil.

Reduce the heat, season with salt and pepper, and then simmer for 15 mins.

Step 5

Turn off the cooker and liquidise with a hand blender. Alternatively pour into a blender machine and blitz until smooth.

Step 6

Mix in the single cream and then serve.

Pea, Leek & Bacon Soup

Ingredients

Servings - 4

2 litres chicken stock (use 2 stock cubes) **Nutrition per serving**

2 medium potatoes, peeled and chopped

2 leeks, chopped

Calories: 289

450g frozen garden peas

Protein: 12g

8 slices of smoked bacon, grilled to crispy   Carbs:

42gchopped into strips

Fat: 8g

Step 1

Cook the 8 slices of bacon under the grill until crispy and set aside.

Step 2

Add the chicken stock cubes to a soup pot and dissolve them with the boiling water.

Step 3

Add in the potatoes and cook for 5 minutes. Next add the sliced leek and let everything boil for 10 minutes.

Step 4

Add in the peas and cook for another 5 mins. Season with salt and pepper then puree everything with a hand blender.

Step 5

Cut the bacon into small strips, mixing the majority of it through and garnishing with a few pieces.

Creamy Carrot & Parsnip Soup

Ingredients

2 tbsp butter

500g carrots, peeled and chopped

2 large parsnips, peeled and chopped

1 large onion, chopped

800ml of vegetable stock

150ml single cream

2 tsp of ground ginger

Grated zest of 1 orange

Salt and pepper

Fresh coriander, to garnish

Servings - 4

Nutrition per serving

Calories: 262

Protein: 4g

Carbs: 30g

Fat: 15g

Step 1

Put a large saucepan on a low heat and melt the butter.

Step 2

Add the chopped onion and cook for 3-4 mins until softened, then add the chopped carrots and parsnips.

Cover the saucepan and cook for 15 minutes, stirring occasionally.

Step 3

Add the ginger, orange zest and stock, then season with salt and pepper.

Step 4

Bring to the boil, then reduce the heat and simmer for 30 minutes until the vegetables are soft.

Step 5

Turn the cooker off and allow the soup to cool for 15 minutes. Then, either using a hand blender or

transferring to a food processor, blitz the soup until smooth.

Step 6

Mix in the cream and, when serving, garnish with fresh coriander.

Salmon Soup

Ingredients

2 tbsp butter

1 leek, sliced

1 large onion, chopped

850ml fish stock

1 large potato, peeled and chopped

1 tbsp plain flour

300g salmon fillets (skin removed),

chopped into small chunks

2 egg yolks

1 tbsp chopped parsley

1 tbsp chopped dill

100ml single cream

Servings - 4

Nutrition per serving:

Calories: 311

Protein: 22g

Carbs: 23g

Fat: 15g

Step 1

Prepare all the vegetables and leave to one side. Add the butter to a large pan and melt over a medium heat.

Step 2

Add the leek and onion and then cook for 3-4 mins on a medium heat until softened.

Step 3

Mix the flour with a little vegetable stock until it makes a paste and then stir into the saucepan.

Step 4

Cook for a couple of minutes and then add in the rest of the vegetable stock, along with the parsley and dill, while stirring throughout.

Step 5

Season with salt and pepper, turn up the heat and then bring to the boil.

Step 6

Reduce the heat and let the soup simmer for 20 mins.

Step 7

Add the salmon chunks and cook for 6-8 mins until cooked through.

Step 8

Whisk together the egg yolks and cream in a bowl, and then stir into the soup. Cook for another 10 mins and then serve.

Creamy Chicken, Bacon & Potato Soup

Ingredients

1 tbsp butter

1 large onion, chopped

3 leeks, sliced and chopped

250g smoked lean bacon, chopped

700g potatoes

2 tbsp plain flour

1 litre chicken stock

3 garlic cloves, chopped

200g skinless chicken breast, diced

4 tbsp double cream

Sea salt and pepper

Fresh parsley

Servings - 4

Nutrition per serving

Calories: 520

Protein: 40g

Carbs: 46g

Fat: 17g

Step 1

Add the butter to a large saucepan and melt over a low heat.

Step 2

Add the onion, leeks and garlic, and cook for 3-4 minutes until softened. Then add in the bacon and allow it to cook through.

Step 3

In a bowl, mix the flour with some of the vegetable stock, enough to make a paste. Stir the paste into the saucepan and then cook for 2-3 minutes, while stirring.

Step 4

Pour in the remaining stock, and add in the potatoes and diced chicken. Season with salt and pepper afterwards.

Step 5

Bring to the boil, then lower the heat and simmer for 25-30 mins until the chicken and potatoes are well cooked.

Step 6

Stir in the double cream and leave to cook for a few more minutes. Meanwhile, grill a slice of bacon until crispy.

Step 7

Serve the soup and garnish with the crispy bacon and parsley.

Mixed Bean Soup

Ingredients

1 tbsp extra virgin olive oil

4 spring onions, chopped

3 garlic cloves, chopped

200g mushrooms, sliced

1 large carrot, peeled and chopped

400g canned mixed beans, drained

800g (2 cans) chopped tomatoes

1 litre vegetable stock

1 tbsp thyme

1 tbsp oregano

4 tbsp double cream

Salt and pepper

Servings - 4

Nutrition per serving

Calories: 262

Protein: 9g

Carbs: 29g

Fat: 13g

Step 1

Add the extra virgin olive oil to a large saucepan and heat at medium.

Step 2

Add the prepared garlic and spring onions, and cook for 3-4 mins until softened.

Step 3

Add the mushrooms, carrots, chopped tomatoes, mixed beans, and vegetable stock.

Step 4

Season with salt and pepper and then bring to the boil.

Step 5

Lower the heat and then simmer for 30 minutes. Then turn off the heat and allow the soup to cool for 15 mins.

Step 6

Either using a hand blender, or by transferring the soup into a food processor, blitz the soup until smooth.

Step 7

Stir in the cream, heat for two more minutes, and then serve.

Split Pea & Courgette Soup

Ingredients

1 large white onion, chopped

2 medium courgettes, diced

200g yellow split peas

1 tbsp extra virgin olive oil

850ml vegetable stock

1/2 tsp turmeric

Sea salt and pepper

Servings - 4

Nutrition per serving

Calories: 153

Protein: 7g

Carbs: 19g

Fat: 5g

Step 1

Put the split peas in a bowl and a pint of water. Allow to soak for a 3-4 hours. Drain the split peas and rinse them before draining again.

Step 2

Add the extra virgin olive oil and heat in a large saucepan at medium.

Step 3

Add in the courgettes and onion, and cook for 3-4 minutes until softened.

Step 4

Pour in the vegetable stock, add the split peas and turmeric, and then bring to the boil.

Step 5

Reduce the heat, season with salt and pepper, and then simmer for 35-40 mins until the split peas are properly cooked through.

Healthy Snacks

- **10 tasty snacks all ridiculously easy to make.**

- **Where protein powder is included in recipes, I recommend <u>plant-based</u> protein (i.e. Sunwarrior or Vegan Blend from MyProtein.com) rather than whey protein powder.**

Nutty Protein Bars

Ingredients	Servings - 5
2 scoops of chocolate protein powder	Nutrition per serving
2 tbsp of oats	
2 tbsp of linseed	Calories: 275
2 handfuls of crushed walnuts	Protein: 22g
2 tablespoons of organic unsweetened peanut butter	Carbs: 13g
4oz (half a glass) of almond milk	Fat: 13g
1 tbsp of Stevia	
1 tsp of cinnamon powder	

Step 1

Add the protein powder, oats, linseed, seeds, Stevia and cinnamon powder to a bowl. Then mix it all up with a spoon. Like a boss.

Step 2

Add the almond milk to moisten the mixture. You may need to add a little more almond milk, but you don't want it to be too runny. Next add in the two tablespoons of peanut butter and stir it thoroughly into the mixture.

Step 3

The peanut butter will help congeal the mixture. Now use your hands to push it all together firmly and roll it into a big ball.

Step 4

Rip chunks of the mixture off the ball and shape them into bars. (You should be able to make 4 decent sized ones with this amount of ingredients).

Step 5

Place them on a foil baking tray and use a little olive oil or butter to grease the bottom so the protein bars don't stick when cooked. Bake at 200°C/400°F/gas 6 for 25-30 mins.

Step 6

Whip your amazing cooking creations out of the oven and smell those little beauties. Forget the fact that they look like baked turds....because they taste awesome.

Coconut Protein Balls

Ingredients

1 cup cashew nuts

1 cup of dates

1 scoop of chocolate protein powder

1 tbsp desiccated coconut

Servings - 6

Nutrition per serving

Calories: 224

Protein: 8g

Carbs: 27g

Fat: 10g

Step 1

For 10 minutes soak the dates in boiling water.

Step 2

Blend the cashew nuts in a food processor.

Step 3

Drain the dates and add them to the food processor with the cashews. Blend until they start to clump together.

Step 4

Next add in the protein powder and blitz until it starts to get crumbly and then clump together again.

Step 5

Roll the mixture into 4 balls with your hands.

Step 6

Scatter the desiccated coconut on parchment paper and roll the balls in it. Place them in a plastic tub and store in the fridge.

Simple Protein Cookies

Ingredients

1 cup oats

2 scoops of chocolate protein powder

1/3 cup unsalted peanuts

1/4 cup coconut oil, melted

2 tbsp unsweetened peanut butter

4 dates, pitted

Cup of water

Servings - 8

Nutrition per serving

Calories: 207

Protein: 9g

Carbs: 12g

Fat: 14g

Step 1

Mix together the oats, peanuts and protein powder in a large mixing bowl.

Step 2

Add the peanut butter, coconut oil, dates and water to a blender and blitz until smooth.

Step 3

Pour this blender mixture into the bowl with the dry ingredients and mix well together. This should be quite thick but add a little more water if there are some dry patches in the bowl.

Step 4

Scoop this cookie mix out onto a chopping board and roll into balls slightly bigger than golf balls, then flatten with your hands.

Step 5

Place the cookies on a baking sheet and put in the fridge for 1 hour to harden before eating.

Sweet As A Nut Balls

Ingredients

1 cup unsweetened almond butter

1/3 cup of coconut cream concentrate melted

3/4 cup of raisins

1/2 cup sunflower seeds

Servings - 8

Nutrition per serving

Calories: 188

Protein: 4g

Carbs: 16g

: 12g

Step 1

Put all ingredients in a food processor and blitz until smooth.

Step 2

Roll into individual balls and place on parchment paper.

Step 3

Place the balls in a plastic tub and refrigerate for 30-60 mins until they harden and are ready to eat.

Choc Coconut Cookie Balls

Ingredients

1/2 cup coconut flour

2 scoops chocolate protein powder

2 tsp baking powder

4 packets Stevia extract

2 tbsp desiccated coconut

1/4 tsp sea salt

1/2 tsp cinnamon

2 egg white

1 tbsp vanilla extract

1/4 cup almond butter

1/4 cup almond milk

1/4 cup mini dark chocolate chips

Servings - 10

Nutrition per serving

Calories: 99

Protein: 7g

Carbs: 6g

Fat: 5g

Step 1

Preheat oven to 180°C/350°F/gas 4. First mix all the dry ingredients in a bowl and then blend in the wet ingredients, mixing with a wooden spoon.

Step 2

Roll into 12 small round balls and place on a baking sheet lined with parchment paper.

Step 3

Bake for 8-10 minutes or until golden brown.

Step 4

Leave to cool for 10 minutes and then serve.

No Bake Brilliant Bars

Ingredients

3 cups of brown rice cereal

2 tbsp honey

2 tbsp unsweetened peanut butter

2 scoops of chocolate protein powder

1/2 cup cashews, crushed

2 tbsp chocolate chips

Servings - 10

Nutrition per serving

Calories: 180

Protein: 8g

Carbs: 22g

Fats: 5g

Step 1

Line a baking tray with parchment paper.

Step 2

Heat a small saucepan on a low heat and add the honey and peanut butter, stirring regularly. Cook for a few minutes until they are melted and well mixed together.

Step 3

Add in the brown rice cereal, protein powder, crushed cashews, and stir everything together for 2-3 minutes. Turn the cooker off and then add in the chocolate chips last (so they don't melt).

Step 4

Using a wooden spoon, transfer the mixture onto the lined baking tray. Place another piece of parchment paper on top and the press down with your hands until the mixture is even as possible.

Step 5

Put in the fridge for 4-5 hours, or overnight, then remove the parchment paper and cut into 10 bars.

Cranberry & Coconut Balls

Ingredients

1/2 cup cranberries

5 medjool dates, pitted

1/2 cup fruit and nut mix

1/2 cup almond flour

1/3 cup coconut flour

2 tbsp chia seeds

2 tbsp coconut oil, melted

2 tbsp honey

2 scoops chocolate or vanilla protein powder

2 tbsp desiccated coconut

Servings - 12

Nutrition per serving

Calories: 168

Protein: 8g

Carbs: 21g

Fat: 7g

Step 1

Add the cranberries, dates, and fruit and nut mix to a food processor and blitz until smooth.

Step 2

Add the almond flour, coconut flour, chia seeds, protein powder, and 1 tbsp of the desiccated coconut and stir together well until the mixture resembles bread crumbs.

Step 3

Add the melted coconut oil, then the honey, and mix well.

Step 4

Roll into 10 small balls using your hands.

Step 5

Spread the remaining desiccated coconut on the kitchen worktop and then roll the balls in it.

Delicious Dates Bites

Ingredients

1 cup of medjool dates, pitted

3/4 cup almonds

3/4 cup walnuts

2 tbsp chia seeds

1 tbsp coconut oil

1 scoop chocolate protein powder

1 tbsp of organic raw cacao powder

Servings - 8

Calories: 246

Protein: 8g

Carbs: 21g

Fat: 17g

Step 1

Add the almonds, walnuts and chia seeds to a food processor and blend until a flour consistency has been created.

Step 2

Add all the remaining ingredients and blend until a sticky dough has formed.

Step 3

Roll the dough into balls, place in a plastic tub, and store in the fridge.

Protein Raisin Cookies

Ingredients

3 scoops chocolate protein powder

200ml canned butter beans

1 tbsp unsweetened natural peanut butter

Handful of raisins

2 tbsp oats

2 tbsp Greek yoghurt

1 tbsp coconut oil

Servings - 6

Nutrition per serving

Calories: 168

Protein: 16g

Carbs: 16g

Fat: 5g

Step 1

Preheat the oven to 150°C/300°F/gas 2.

Step 2

Add all ingredients in a blender and blitz until blend until a dough is created. If too dry, add a little almond milk or another tbsp of yoghurt.

Step 3

Separate the dough into six balls and flatten with the palms of your hands.

Step 4

Place some parchment paper in a baking tin and add the cookies. Cook in the oven for 10-12 minutes or until golden brown.

Almond Fudge Bars

Ingredients   Servings - 6

2 scoops vanilla or chocolate protein powder

Nutrition per serving

1.5 cup oats

2 tbsp almond butter   Calories: 233

2 tbsp honey   Protein: 13g

1 cup Rice Crispies cereal   Carbs: 36g

1 tsp vanilla extract   Fat: 5g

2 tbsp almond milk

Step 1

Add a sheet of parchment paper to a casserole dish / baking tray.

Step 2

Grind 1 cup of oats into a flour consistency and then add to a large mixing bowl, along with another 1/2 cup of oats, protein powder and Rice Crispies cereal.

Step 3

Put a small saucepan on a low-medium heat and melt the almond butter. Then mix in the honey and vanilla extract, stirring for 2-3 mins.

Step 4

Remove from the heat and add to the other ingredients in the mixing bowl, stirring well until they are combined.

Step 5

Using a wooden spoon, transfer the mixture into the cooking dish / baking tray and flatten in evenly with the palms of your hands.

Step 6

Place in the fridge for 45-60 mins and then cut into separate bars.

Healthy Shakes

- A blender (not a juicer) is essential. You can find a decent one online via Amazon for around £30.

- Simply chuck all ingredients in these recipes in blender and blitz for 1 minute until smooth.

- The first three recipes are intentionally higher in calories for people looking to gain weight and muscle mass
(instructions are also provided to reduce the calorie count).

- Again, I recommend plant-based protein powders (i.e. Sunwarrior or Vegan Blend from MyProtein.com)
rather than whey protein powder with these recipes.

Blueberry Blast

Ingredients	Nutrition per shake
Handful of frozen blueberries	Calories: 850
1/2 ripe banana	Protein: 30g
1 scoop of chocolate protein powder	Carbs: 73g
Half tin (200ml) coconut milk	Fat: 49g
2 tbsp oats	
1/4 tsp cinnamon	
Cup of water	
2 or 3 ice cubes	

(Using only 1/4 tin of coconut milk instead will reduce the calories by around 150-170).

Choc n' Banana

Ingredients

1 ripe banana

1 scoop choc protein powder

1 tbsp unsweetened peanut butter

Handful of almonds / mixed nuts

1 tbsp oats

1 tbsp linseed

1/4 tsp cinnamon

Cup of water

2 or 3 ice cubes

Nutrition per shake

Calories: 685

Protein: 40g

Carbs: 58g

Fat: 33g

(Using only 1 tbsp of peanut butter will reduce calories by 100-150).

Mango Monster

Ingredients

1 cup of frozen mango

1 scoop of chocolate protein powder

Half can (200ml) coconut milk

2 tbsp linseed

2 tbsp sunflower seeds

1/4 tsp ginger and/or nutmeg

Handful of spinach

Cup of water

2 or 3 ice cubes

Nutrition per shake

Calories: 900

Protein: 39g

Carbs: 33g

Fat: 69g

* (Using only 1/4 tin of coconut milk will reduce the calories by around 150-170).

Avocado Attack

Ingredients

2 tbsp of oats

Half an avocado

Handful of pumpkin seeds

1 tbsp of peanut butter

1 scoop of protein powder

1-1.5 cups of water

Nutrition per shake

Calories: 600

Protein: 37g

Carbs: 42g

Fat: 32g

Strawberry Goji Smooth

Ingredients

Nutrition per shake

1 scoops of strawberry protein powder   Calories: 262

2 cups of unsweetened almond milk (or water)

Protein: 18g

3 fresh strawberries   Carbs: 24g

1-2 tsp goji powder   Fat: 9g

2 or 3 ice cubes

Tropical Twist

Ingredients

1 scoop of vanilla or plain protein powder

1/4 cup frozen pineapple chunks

1/2 frozen banana

1/2 cup frozen mango chunks

1 cup of almond milk (or water)

2 or 3 ice cubes

Nutrition per shake

Calories: 220

Protein: 28g

Carbs: 53g

Fat: 7g

Green Pineapple Power

Ingredients

½ cup unsweetened almond milk

⅓ cup nonfat plain Greek yogurt

1 cup baby spinach

1 frozen banana

½ cup frozen pineapple chunks

1 tablespoon chia seeds

1-2 tsps of honey

Nutrition per shake

Calories: 420

Protein: 12g

Carbs: 55g

Fat: 18g

Ginger Booster

Ingredients

200g Greek natural yoghurt

1 frozen banana

2 tbsp almond butter

1 tsp ground ginger

1/4 tsp ground cinnamon

Cup of water

2 or 3 ice cubes

Nutrition per shake

Calories: 528

Protein: 17g

Carbs: 41g

Fat: 35g

Chia Berry

Ingredients

200g Greek natural yoghurt

1 frozen banana

100g blueberries

3 or 4 large strawberries

1/4 tsp ground ginger

Cup of water

2 or 3 ice cubes

Nutrition per shake

Calories: 422

Protein: 11g

Carbs: 54g

Fat: 20g

Tropical Treat

Ingredients

1 scoop vanilla protein powder

300ml pineapple juice

1/2 frozen banana

2 tbsp Greek yoghurt

3 or 4 large strawberries

2 or 3 ice cubes

Nutrition per shake

Calories: 336

Protein: 12g

Carbs: 58g

Fat: 7g

About the author

Marc McLean is a 30 something year old online personal training and nutrition coach from Loch Lomond in Scotland. He owns Weight Training Is The Way and is a health and fitness writer for leading websites including The Good Men Project, Mind Body Green, and Healthgreatness.com

Marc is the author of the Strength Training 101 series on Amazon, which also includes:

* *Strength Training Program 101: Build Muscle & Burn Fat...In Less Than 3 Hours Per Week.*

* *Strength Training For Women: Burn Fat Effectively...And Sculpt The Body You've Always Dreamed Of*

Marc loves...climbing Munros (aka the biggest hills) in Scotland, peanut butter, amazing scenery, the Rocky movies, lifting heavy things, blueberries, Daft Punk, watching tennis, travelling and laughing. Not in that particular order.

Marc hates...bad manners, funerals, cardio, and all drivers who don't indicate.

You can connect with Marc here:

Email: marc@weighttrainingistheway.com

Website: www.weighttrainingistheway.com

Facebook: www.facebook.com/weighttrainingistheway

Instagram: www.instagram.com/weight_training_is_the_way

Made in the USA
Middletown, DE
23 April 2019